# Unbreakable
# Mastering Chronic Pain
# Management for a Limitless Life

Wendy Sauer & Amy Rached

# Dedication

To all those living with chronic pain, this book is dedicated to you.

May it provide you with knowledge and strategies to help manage your pain and improve your quality of life.

May it remind you that you are not alone in your journey and that there is hope for a better tomorrow.

May you find the resilience and courage to face the challenges ahead and the inspiration to live a fulfilling and meaningful life.

This book is for you, dear readers, with the utmost respect and admiration for your strength and perseverance.

Dedication is a quality that is often lauded but seldom truly understood. To dedicate oneself is to commit oneself wholly to a cause or purpose without reserve or hesitation. It is to set aside personal concerns and ambition to pursue a greater goal. In short, it is the opposite of selfishness.

Those who dedicate their lives to others – whether it be their families, their communities, or humanity as a whole – are the true heroes of our world. They are the ones who make sacrifices for the greater good, who put others before themselves, and who never give up even when the odds are against them.

So today, I want to take a moment to pay tribute to those who have dedicated their lives to helping others. Unfortunately, it is rare to find compassion and a proper grasp of human nature amongst those who practice science and medicine. However, there are a few exceptions to this rule.

Dr Allan Bartlett has cared for 4 generations of my family and has always provided excellent care due to his vast medical knowledge and experience. Dr Emile Malek has also been a fabulous family practitioner, and his dedication to his elderly patients and his practice is admirable and exceptional. Last but not least, Dr John Arbuckle has been a constant source of support and guidance, always offering outstanding care and inspiring advice on antiaging strategies, scientific updates, and medical breakthroughs, rescuing us when we need it most.

These three men have been an integral part of our lives, and we are forever grateful for their compassion and expertise. We dedicate this book to them in hopes that it will inspire others in their fields of medicine and science to follow in their footsteps.

# About this book

Chronic pain can be an incredibly isolating experience. Many people feel trapped in a cycle of pain, medication, and immobility that leaves them feeling defeated and disconnected from society. If you're living with chronic pain, you may be wondering where to turn for help and how to take your next steps towards wellness.

The truth is, there is always a better way. The key to overcoming chronic pain is learning how to communicate with your body in a new way. It may be a process full of repetition and hard work, but the results are worth it. With the right tools and techniques, you can break free from the cycle of pain and take control of your life.

This is where our book comes in. It offers a comprehensive guide to understanding chronic pain and provides practical strategies for managing and reducing pain levels. Our expert authors draw from years of experience in pain management to offer you a revolutionary approach to healing from chronic pain.

Through targeted exercises, stretches, and mindfulness practices, you'll learn how to communicate with your body and break free from the cycle of pain. You'll discover how to address the root causes of your pain and take proactive steps towards improving your physical, emotional, and mental wellbeing.

If you're tired of feeling defeated by chronic pain and want to take control of your life, our book is the perfect resource for you. With our guidance, you can learn how to build new neural pathways and create a life full of joy, movement, and possibility. Don't let chronic pain hold you back any longer – start your journey towards healing today.

# Table of Contents

Dedication ................................................................................................ 2
About this book ...................................................................................... 5
Table of Contents .................................................................................... 7
COPYRIGHT ............................................................................................ 10
Introduction ........................................................................................... 11
    Explanation of what chronic pain is and how it affects people's lives ............... 12
    Importance of taking control of chronic pain ............................................ 15
    Purpose of the book and what readers can expect to gain from it .................. 18
Chapter 1 ............................................................................................... 19
Understanding Chronic Pain & The Science of Chronic Pain ............... 19
    Overview of the anatomy and physiology of pain ...................................... 20
    Explanation of how chronic pain differs from acute pain ............................. 22
    **Understanding the types and causes of chronic pain** ............................. 24
    Explanation of how chronic pain can affect mental health and overall wellbeing ............................................................................................................. 26
Chapter 2 Diagnosis and Treatment ..................................................... 35
    Treatment of Chronic Pain ................................................................... 38
    Understanding how chronic pain is diagnosed ......................................... 39
    Overview of different treatment options, such as medication, physical therapy, and alternative therapies .................................................................... 41
    Explanation of how to work with healthcare providers to create a personalized treatment plan .................................................................................. 68
    Strategies for finding and working with a pain management team ............... 70
Chapter 3 ............................................................................................... 72
The Role of Lifestyle Changes in Managing Chronic Pain .................... 72
    Overview of Lifestyle Changes for Chronic Pain Management ..................... 72

- Implementing Lifestyle Changes for Chronic Pain Management ......... 73
- Explanation of how lifestyle changes can affect chronic pain ............ 74
- Tips for creating a supportive and safe environment for rehabilitation ............ 76
- Strategies for adopting healthy habits such as nutrition, exercise, and sleep .. 77
- Tips for creating a supportive and safe environment for rehabilitation ............ 79
- Ways to integrate relaxation techniques into daily life ......... 89

Chapter 4 ......... 93

Mind-Body Techniques for Managing Chronic Pain ......... 93

- Overview of mind-body techniques such as mindfulness, meditation, and cognitive-behavioural therapy ......... 94
- Explanation of how these techniques can help manage chronic pain and improve mental health ......... 99

Tips for integrating mind-body techniques into daily life and treatment plans .... 102

Real-life examples of successful mind-body techniques ......... 105

Chapter 5 Coping Strategies ......... 106

- Strategies for coping with the emotional and psychological impact of chronic pain ......... 107
- How to build a support network of family, friends, and healthcare providers .. 111
- Tips for managing stress, anxiety, and depression ......... 112
- The importance of self-care and self-compassion ......... 114

Chapter 6: Advanced Pain Management Techniques ......... 134

- Explanation of advanced pain management techniques such as nerve blocks, spinal cord stimulation, and infusion therapy ......... 138
- How these techniques can be used to manage chronic pain ......... 141
- What to expect during advanced pain management procedures ......... 146
- Potential risks and benefits of advanced pain management techniques ......... 148

Chapter 7 Strategies for Long-Term Success ......... 154

Understanding how to maintain progress and continue managing chronic pain in the long term.................................................................................................165

Strategies for preventing relapse and managing setbacks...............................167

Tips for adjusting to life with chronic pain and finding meaning and purpose.170

The importance of resilience and cultivating a positive mindset.......................175

Conclusion: ......................................................................................................177

Recap of key points and takeaways from the book ..........................................178

Final words of encouragement and inspiration for readers to take control of their chronic pain and improve their quality of life.............................................179

## COPYRIGHT

Copyright © 2023 by Wendy Sauer http://www.smashchronicpain.com

All rights reserved. This book or any part thereof may not be reproduced or used in any manner whatsoever without the publisher's express written permission except for the use of brief quotations in a book review.

This book is not intended as a substitute for the medical recommendations of physicians, mental health professionals, or other healthcare providers. Rather, it is intended to offer information to help the reader cooperate with their physicians, mental health professionals, and healthcare providers in a mutual quest for optimal well-being.

# Introduction

Greetings, dear reader! Welcome to this light-hearted exploration of a topic that affects many of us: chronic pain. While this may seem like a heavy and daunting subject, I assure you that we will approach it with a sense of curiosity, openness, and even a touch of humour.

Firstly, let's acknowledge that chronic pain is a real and challenging condition that affects millions of people worldwide. Whether you are dealing with chronic pain yourself or you know someone who is, it can be a difficult and isolating experience. But the good news is that there are ways to manage chronic pain and improve your quality of life.

Throughout this book, we'll explore the science behind chronic pain, the various treatment options available, and the lifestyle changes and coping strategies that can help you live a fulfilling life despite chronic pain. We'll also delve into some of the more advanced techniques and cutting-edge research in the field of pain management.

Now, I understand that this may sound like a dry academic text but fear not! I promise to keep things engaging and even a bit light hearted. After all, humour can be a powerful tool in managing chronic pain and coping with the challenges it presents. So, get ready to learn, laugh, and conquer chronic pain together. Let us get started!

Explanation of what chronic pain is and how it affects people's lives

Chronic pain is a complex and multifaceted condition that affects millions of people worldwide. It is defined as pain that lasts for at least three months or longer, beyond the typical healing period of an injury or illness. Chronic pain can be caused by a wide range of underlying conditions, including arthritis, back pain, fibromyalgia, nerve damage, and cancer, among others.

Chronic pain can take many forms, ranging from a persistent ache to a sharp or shooting pain that comes and goes. It can also manifest as a burning, tingling, or numb sensation, and may be accompanied by other symptoms such as fatigue, sleep disturbances, and mood changes.

While acute pain serves a protective function and is a necessary response to injury or illness, chronic pain is not helpful or necessary for healing. In fact, chronic pain can be a sign that something is wrong in the body and can be a challenging and debilitating experience for those who live with it.

The impact of chronic pain on people's lives is significant and far-reaching. It can affect physical, emotional, and social well-being, and can have a ripple effect on every aspect of daily life. Chronic pain can limit mobility and interfere with activities of daily living, such as walking, bending, or standing. It can also impact the ability to work or engage in hobbies and interests, leading to feelings of frustration, isolation, and boredom.

Chronic pain can also have a significant impact on mental health, contributing to the development of anxiety, depression, and other mood disorders. Living with chronic pain can lead to feelings of hopelessness, anger, and despair, and can impact overall quality of life.

One of the most challenging aspects of chronic pain is its unpredictability. Pain levels can fluctuate from day to day, or even from hour to hour, making it difficult to plan and manage daily activities. This uncertainty can lead to feelings of anxiety and stress and can make it difficult to maintain social relationships and engage in meaningful activities.

Despite its challenges, it's important to remember that chronic pain is a real and valid experience that deserves attention and care. With the right treatment and support, people with chronic pain can learn to manage their symptoms, improve their overall health and well-being, and live a fulfilling life.

In recent years, there has been a growing recognition of the importance of a holistic approach to chronic pain management. This approach recognizes that chronic pain is not just a physical experience, but also has emotional, social, and psychological components. As a result, effective chronic pain management often involves a combination of medical interventions, lifestyle modifications, and emotional and psychological support.

Medical interventions for chronic pain can include medications, physical therapy, and alternative therapies such as acupuncture or massage. These interventions can help manage pain levels, improve mobility, and function, and prevent further injury or damage.

Lifestyle modifications are also an important aspect of chronic pain management. This can include adopting a healthy diet, regular exercise, and stress management techniques such as mindfulness or meditation. These lifestyle changes can help improve overall health and wellbeing and can also reduce pain levels and improve function.

Emotional and psychological support is also an essential component of chronic pain management. This can include counselling or therapy to help manage stress, anxiety, and depression, as well as support groups or peer counselling to provide a sense of community and support.

While chronic pain can be a challenging and difficult experience, it's important to remember that there are effective treatments and strategies for managing pain and improving quality of life. With the right support and guidance, people with chronic pain can learn to live well and thrive despite their pain.

Importance of taking control of chronic pain

Taking control of chronic pain is an essential aspect of managing the condition and improving overall quality of life. While chronic pain can be a complex and challenging experience, there are effective strategies and treatments that can help reduce pain levels, improve function and mobility, and enhance overall health and well-being.

One of the most important reasons to take control of chronic pain is to prevent further damage or injury. Chronic pain can lead to changes in posture, movement patterns, and activity levels, which can further exacerbate pain levels and increase the risk of injury. By taking control of chronic pain, people can work with healthcare providers and pain management specialists to identify underlying conditions, develop personalized treatment plans, and learn strategies for managing pain levels and preventing further damage.

Taking control of chronic pain can also help improve physical function and mobility. Chronic pain can limit movement and activity levels, which can lead to muscle weakness, stiffness, and reduced range of motion. By working with healthcare providers and pain management specialists, people with chronic pain can learn exercises and techniques to improve strength, flexibility, and mobility, which can enhance overall physical function and reduce the risk of further injury.

In addition to physical function, taking control of chronic pain can also improve emotional and psychological well-being. Chronic pain can lead to feelings of anxiety, depression, and social isolation, which can further exacerbate pain levels and impact overall quality of life. By taking control of chronic pain, people can work with mental health professionals and support groups to learn coping strategies, develop a sense of community, and enhance overall emotional and psychological well-being.

Another important reason to take control of chronic pain is to improve overall health and well-being. Chronic pain can have a significant impact on physical health, leading to sleep disturbances, poor nutrition, and increased risk of other health conditions. By taking control of chronic pain, people can work with healthcare providers and pain management specialists to address underlying health conditions, develop healthy lifestyle habits, and improve overall health and well-being.

Taking control of chronic pain can also improve social well-being and quality of life. Chronic pain can limit social activities and engagement, leading to feelings of isolation and disconnection. By taking control of chronic pain, people can learn social strategies and techniques to enhance social support and engagement, develop a sense of community, and improve overall quality of life.

One of the most important aspects of taking control of chronic pain is the recognition that people with chronic pain are not alone. Chronic pain is a common experience that affects millions of people worldwide, and there is a growing community of healthcare providers, pain management

specialists, and support groups that can provide guidance, supp
resources for managing pain and improving quality of life.

Taking control of chronic pain requires a multifaceted approach that recognizes the physical, emotional, and social components of the condition. This approach may involve medical interventions, lifestyle modifications, and emotional and psychological support, depending on the individual's needs and preferences.

Medical interventions for chronic pain may include medications, physical therapy, and alternative therapies such as acupuncture or massage. These interventions can help manage pain levels, improve mobility, and function, and prevent further injury or damage.

Lifestyle modifications are also an important aspect of chronic pain management. This may include adopting a healthy diet, regular exercise, and stress management techniques such as mindfulness or meditation. These lifestyle changes can help improve overall health and well-being and can also reduce pain levels and improve function.

Emotional and psychological support is also an essential component of chronic pain management. This may include counselling or therapy to help manage stress, anxiety, and depression, as well as support groups or peer counselling to provide a sense of community and support.

Purpose of the book and what readers can expect to gain from it

The purpose of this book is to provide a comprehensive guide for people living with chronic pain, their loved ones, and healthcare providers. This book aims to provide a practical and holistic approach to chronic pain management, incorporating medical interventions, lifestyle modifications, and emotional and psychological support.

Readers can expect to gain a deeper understanding of what chronic pain is and how it affects people's lives. This book will provide insights into the underlying causes of chronic pain, the different types of chronic pain, and the common symptoms associated with chronic pain. Readers will also learn about the various medical interventions available for managing chronic pain, including medications, physical therapy, and alternative therapies.

In addition to medical interventions, readers can expect to gain insights into the importance of lifestyle modifications for managing chronic pain. This book will provide practical tips and strategies for adopting healthy habits such as nutrition, exercise, and sleep, as well as relaxation techniques such as meditation and mindfulness.

Furthermore, readers can expect to learn about the importance of emotional and psychological support for managing chronic pain. This book will explore the impact of chronic pain on mental health, including the development of anxiety, depression, and other mood disorders. Readers will also gain insights into the various emotional and psychological support options available, such as counselling, therapy, and support groups.

By the end of this book, readers can expect to have a comprehensive understanding of chronic pain, as well as the tools and strategies needed to manage the condition effectively. They will learn how to work with healthcare providers and pain management specialists to create a personalized treatment plan, adopt healthy lifestyle habits, and develop coping strategies to improve their overall quality of life. Whether you are living with chronic pain or supporting someone who is, this book is designed to provide practical and actionable advice for taking control of chronic pain and improving your overall well-being.

# Chapter 1

Understanding Chronic Pain & The Science of Chronic Pain

Overview of the anatomy and physiology of pain
Understanding the anatomy and physiology of pain is essential for anyone living with chronic pain, as it can help provide insights into the underlying causes and potential treatment options. Pain is a complex and multifaceted experience that involves a range of physiological processes,

from the initial injury or damage to the transmission of signals through the nervous system and the processing of those signals in the brain.

The anatomy of pain can be broken down into three main components: nociceptors, nerves, and the brain. Nociceptors are specialized nerve cells that detect and respond to noxious stimuli, such as heat, pressure, or chemical irritants. These nociceptors are located throughout the body, including the skin, muscles, bones, and organs.

When nociceptors are activated by a noxious stimulus, they send electrical signals through nerves to the spinal cord, where the signals are processed and transmitted to the brain. The spinal cord acts as a relay centre, sending signals up to the brain and receiving signals back down to the muscles and organs.

The brain plays a crucial role in the experience of pain, as it is responsible for processing and interpreting the signals received from the spinal cord. Different areas of the brain are involved in different aspects of pain processing, such as the sensory aspects of pain, the emotional response to pain, and the cognitive appraisal of pain.

The physiology of pain is equally complex, involving a range of neurotransmitters, hormones, and other signalling molecules that influence the experience of pain. When nociceptors are activated, they release chemicals such as prostaglandins, histamines, and cytokines, which can sensitize nearby nerves and increase the intensity of pain signals.

In addition to these chemicals, there are a range of neurotransmitters that are involved in pain processing, including substance P, glutamate, and endorphins. Substance P is involved in the transmission of pain signals from the periphery to the spinal cord, while glutamate is involved in the transmission of pain signals from the spinal cord to the brain. Endorphins, on the other hand, are natural painkillers that are released in response to pain and can help reduce the intensity of pain signals.

The physiology of pain is also influenced by a range of hormones, including cortisol, adrenaline, and testosterone. Cortisol is a stress hormone that can increase pain sensitivity, while adrenaline can increase heart rate and blood pressure, making the experience of pain more intense. Testosterone, on the other hand, has been shown to have analgesic effects, reducing the intensity of pain signals.

Understanding the anatomy and physiology of pain is essential for effective pain management, as it can help healthcare providers and pain management specialists identify underlying causes, develop personalized treatment plans, and determine the most appropriate interventions for managing pain. By taking a comprehensive and holistic approach to pain management, people living with chronic pain can learn to take control of their condition and improve their overall quality of life.

Explanation of how chronic pain differs from acute pain

Chronic pain and acute pain are two different types of pain that are characterized by their duration and underlying causes. While acute pain is a normal and necessary response to injury or illness, chronic pain is a persistent, long-lasting pain that can last for months, years, or even a lifetime.

Acute pain is a type of pain that typically lasts for a short period of time and is usually caused by an injury or illness. Acute pain is a normal and necessary response to injury or illness, as it helps to protect the body and prevent further damage. For example, if you sprain your ankle, you may experience acute pain that lasts for a few days or weeks, but as the injury heals, the pain subsides.

Chronic pain, on the other hand, is a type of pain that persists beyond the typical healing period of an injury or illness. Chronic pain can be caused by a wide range of underlying conditions, including arthritis, back pain, fibromyalgia, nerve damage, and cancer, among others. Unlike acute pain, which serves a protective function and is a necessary response to injury or illness, chronic pain is not helpful or necessary for healing.

One of the key differences between acute and chronic pain is their duration. Acute pain typically lasts for a brief period of time, ranging from a few days to a few weeks, while chronic pain persists beyond the typical healing period and can last for months, years, or even a lifetime.

Another difference between acute and chronic pain is their intensity. Acute pain is often described as sharp or intense, and can be associated with swelling, redness, or other signs of inflammation. Chronic pain, on the other hand, may be less intense but can be persistent and difficult to manage. Chronic pain can also be associated with other symptoms, such as fatigue, sleep disturbances, and mood changes.

The impact of acute and chronic pain on people's lives can also differ. Acute pain is usually a temporary inconvenience that can be managed with rest, medication, or other interventions. Chronic pain, on the other hand, can have a significant impact on physical, emotional, and social well-being, and can limit mobility, interfere with daily activities, and impact the ability to work or engage in hobbies and interests.

In summary, acute pain is a short-term response to injury or illness that serves a protective function, while chronic pain is a persistent, long-lasting pain that can have a significant impact on physical, emotional, and social well-being. Understanding the differences between these two types of pain is essential for effective pain management and improving quality of life for people living with chronic pain.

**Understanding the types and causes of chronic pain**

Chronic pain is a complex and multifaceted condition that can be caused by a wide range of underlying conditions. Understanding the types and causes of chronic pain is essential for effective pain management and improving quality of life for people living with this condition.

There are several different types of chronic pain, including neuropathic pain, nociceptive pain, and psychogenic pain. Neuropathic pain is caused by damage to the nerves, such as from injuries or illnesses like diabetes, multiple sclerosis, or shingles. Nociceptive pain, on the other hand, is caused by tissue damage, such as from arthritis, back pain, or fibromyalgia. Psychogenic pain is caused by psychological or emotional factors, such as stress, depression, or anxiety.

The underlying causes of chronic pain can be divided into several categories, including musculoskeletal, neurological, visceral, and idiopathic causes. Musculoskeletal causes of chronic pain include conditions like arthritis, back pain, and fibromyalgia. Neurological causes include conditions like neuropathy, multiple sclerosis, and strokes. Visceral causes of chronic pain include conditions like endometriosis, irritable bowel syndrome, and interstitial cystitis. Idiopathic causes of chronic pain are those that are not well understood and may have no identifiable underlying cause.

One of the most common causes of chronic pain is musculoskeletal conditions, such as arthritis and back pain. Arthritis is a condition that causes inflammation of the joints, leading to pain, swelling, and stiffness. Back pain is a common condition that can be caused by a range of underlying conditions, including herniated discs, spinal stenosis, or muscle strain.

Neuropathic pain is another common cause of chronic pain, particularly in people with conditions like diabetes or multiple sclerosis. Neuropathy can cause numbness, tingling, or burning sensations, as well as shooting or stabbing pain.

Visceral pain is often caused by conditions affecting the internal organs, such as endometriosis, irritable bowel syndrome, or interstitial cystitis. These conditions can cause pain and discomfort in the abdomen, pelvis, or urinary tract.

In some cases, chronic pain may have no identifiable underlying cause, which can make it particularly challenging to manage. This is known as idiopathic pain and may require a more comprehensive and holistic approach to pain management, incorporating lifestyle modifications, psychological support, and alternative therapies.

Explanation of how chronic pain can affect mental health and overall wellbeing

Chronic pain can have a significant impact on mental health and overall well-being. Living with persistent pain can be challenging and can lead to a range of emotional and psychological symptoms, including anxiety, depression, anger, frustration, and social isolation.

One of the ways in which chronic pain can affect mental health is by leading to the development of anxiety and depression. Chronic pain can cause individuals to feel helpless, hopeless, and out of control, which can lead to the development of anxiety and depression. These mental health conditions can exacerbate the pain, creating a vicious cycle of pain and negative emotions.

Chronic pain can also interfere with sleep, which can have a significant impact on mental health and overall well-being. Poor sleep quality and insomnia are common among individuals living with chronic pain, which can lead to fatigue, irritability, and difficulty concentrating. Sleep disturbance can also exacerbate pain, making it even more challenging to manage.

In addition to the direct impact on mental health, chronic pain can also have an indirect impact on overall well-being. People living with chronic pain may find that they are unable to participate in activities that they enjoy, leading to feelings of social isolation and a loss of purpose. Chronic pain can also interfere with work, leading to financial stress and reduced quality of life.

Furthermore, the use of pain medications to manage chronic pain can also have a range of side effects, including drowsiness, nausea, and constipation. These side effects can impact daily life and further contribute to the negative impact of chronic pain on mental health and overall well-being.

Overall, chronic pain can have a significant impact on mental health and overall well-being. It is important for healthcare providers and pain management specialists to take a comprehensive and holistic approach to pain management, incorporating psychological support and emotional counselling to help individuals living with chronic pain cope with the emotional and psychological impact of their condition. By addressing both the physical and emotional aspects of chronic pain, individuals can improve their overall quality of life and better manage their condition. When it comes to chronic pain, there are both psychosocial and physiological considerations to take into account.

Psychosocial factors refer to the psychological and social factors that can influence pain perception and management. These factors can include stress, anxiety, depression, social support, and beliefs and attitudes about pain. Research has shown that these factors can significantly impact the experience of pain and addressing them can be an important part of a pain management program.

For example, stress and anxiety can lead to increased muscle tension and pain, while social support can help reduce the emotional and physical burden of pain. Cognitive-behavioral therapy, mindfulness meditation, and relaxation techniques are all examples of psychosocial interventions that can be used to address these factors.

Physiological factors refer to the biological processes that can contribute to pain, such as inflammation, nerve damage, and changes in the central nervous system. These factors can often be addressed through medical interventions, such as medication, physical therapy, and surgery.

However, it is important to note that psychosocial and physiological factors are often interconnected and addressing one can impact the other. For example, reducing stress and anxiety through psychosocial interventions can lead to a reduction in inflammation and pain.

Therefore, a comprehensive pain management program should address both psychosocial and physiological factors to achieve the best outcomes for the individual. This may involve a multidisciplinary approach, including healthcare providers such as doctors, physical therapists, psychologists, and nutritionists, working together to develop an individualized plan for managing pain.

Chronic pain is a complex condition that can have a significant impact on an individual's physical, emotional, and social well-being. Therefore, a comprehensive approach that takes into account the multiple factors that contribute to chronic pain is needed to manage the condition effectively.

Psychosocial Considerations:

Psychosocial factors are the psychological and social factors that can influence pain perception and management. These factors can include stress, anxiety, depression, social support, and beliefs and attitudes about pain.

1. Stress:

Stress can have a significant impact on chronic pain. Stress can increase muscle tension and lead to the release of stress hormones that can worsen inflammation and pain. Furthermore, the anticipation of pain can increase stress levels and worsen pain perception.

Psychosocial interventions, such as cognitive-behavioral therapy, mindfulness meditation, and relaxation techniques, can help individuals reduce stress levels and improve pain management.

2. Anxiety and Depression:

Anxiety and depression are common among individuals with chronic pain. These conditions can worsen pain perception and lead to decreased quality of life.

Psychosocial interventions, such as cognitive-behavioral therapy and acceptance and commitment therapy, can help individuals address anxiety and depression and improve pain management.

3. Social Support:

Social support can help individuals with chronic pain manage the emotional and physical burden of pain. Social support can come from family, friends, support groups, and healthcare providers.

Social support can also help individuals feel less isolated and provide opportunities for socialization and physical activity.

4. Beliefs and Attitudes About Pain:

Beliefs and attitudes about pain can significantly impact pain perception and management. For example, individuals who believe that pain is a sign of weakness may be less likely to seek treatment for their pain.

Cognitive-behavioral therapy can help individuals address negative beliefs and attitudes about pain and improve pain management.

Physiological Considerations:

Physiological factors are the biological processes that can contribute to pain, such as inflammation, nerve damage, and changes in the central nervous system.

1. Inflammation:

Inflammation is a common cause of chronic pain. Inflammation can occur due to injury, infection, or chronic health conditions such as arthritis.

Medical interventions, such as nonsteroidal anti-inflammatory drugs (NSAIDs) and corticosteroids, can help reduce inflammation and improve pain management.

2. Nerve Damage:

Nerve damage can result in chronic pain conditions such as neuropathic pain. Nerve damage can occur due to injury, infection, or chronic health conditions such as diabetes.

Medical interventions, such as nerve blocks and medication such as gabapentin and pregabalin, can help reduce nerve-related pain.

3. Changes in the Central Nervous System:

Chronic pain can lead to changes in the central nervous system that can worsen pain perception. These changes can include alterations in the way pain signals are processed and changes in the structure and function of the brain.

Medical interventions, such as medication and cognitive-behavioral therapy, can help address changes in the central nervous system and improve pain management.

Comprehensive Pain Management:

A comprehensive approach to pain management involves addressing both psychosocial and physiological factors that contribute to chronic pain. This may involve a multidisciplinary approach, including healthcare providers such as doctors, physical therapists, psychologists, and nutritionists, working together to develop an individualized plan for managing pain.

The following are some of the components of a comprehensive pain management program:

1. Medication:

Medication is often an important component of pain management. Medication can help reduce inflammation, nerve-related pain, and pain perception.

However, medication should be used judiciously and under the guidance of a healthcare provider to minimize side

effects and potential risks. Medication should also be combined with other pain management strategies for the best outcomes.

2. Physical Therapy:

Physical therapy can help individuals with chronic pain improve their physical functioning and reduce pain. Physical therapy can involve exercise, manual therapy, and other modalities.

Physical therapy can also help individuals address muscle weakness, joint stiffness, and other physical limitations that can contribute to chronic pain.

3. Cognitive-Behavioral Therapy:

Cognitive-behavioral therapy (CBT) can help individuals with chronic pain address negative beliefs and attitudes about pain and improve pain management. CBT can also help individuals address anxiety and depression, which are common among individuals with chronic pain.

CBT involves identifying and challenging negative thoughts and behaviours related to pain and developing coping strategies to manage pain.

4. Mindfulness-Based Interventions:

Mindfulness-based interventions, such as mindfulness-based stress reduction and mindfulness-based cognitive therapy, can help individuals with chronic pain reduce stress and improve pain management.

These interventions involve learning mindfulness techniques, such as meditation and body scanning, to improve awareness of the present moment and reduce stress.

5. Nutrition:

Nutrition can also play a role in chronic pain management. A diet rich in whole foods, fruits, vegetables, lean proteins, and healthy fats can provide the necessary nutrients and antioxidants to support the immune system and reduce inflammation.

On the other hand, a diet high in processed and sugary foods can increase inflammation and pain. Nutrition should be combined with other pain management strategies for the best outcomes.

6. Sleep:

Sleep is an important component of pain management. Lack of sleep can worsen pain perception and lead to increased stress levels.

Sleep hygiene practices, such as establishing a regular sleep schedule, avoiding caffeine and alcohol, and creating a relaxing sleep environment, can improve sleep quality and reduce pain perception.

Chronic pain is a complex condition that requires a comprehensive approach to management. Psychosocial and physiological factors can significantly impact pain perception and management, and addressing both of these factors is important for improving pain outcomes.

# Chapter 2 Diagnosis and Treatment

To get the best outcomes from your treatment and management of chronic pain, it is important to take a proactive approach and be actively involved in your care. Here are some steps you can take to get the best outcomes from your treatment:

1. Be Honest and Open with Your Healthcare Providers:

Be honest and open with your healthcare providers about your pain and any other symptoms or concerns you may have. Provide them with as much information as possible about your pain, including when it started, what makes it better or worse, and how it affects your daily life.

2. Ask Questions:

Don't be afraid to ask questions about your pain, diagnosis, and treatment options. Ask your healthcare providers to explain any medical terms or procedures that you don't understand. This can help you make informed decisions about your care.

3. Follow Treatment Plans:

Follow the treatment plan recommended by your healthcare providers, including medication, physical therapy, and other interventions. It is important to be consistent with your treatment plan and attend all scheduled appointments.

4. Practice Self-Care:

In addition to following your treatment plan, practice self-care by taking care of your physical and emotional well-being. This may include eating a healthy diet, exercising regularly, getting enough sleep, and practicing stress-reducing techniques such as mindfulness or meditation.

5. Track Your Progress:

Keep track of your pain levels, medication usage, and any changes in your symptoms. This can help you and your healthcare providers evaluate the effectiveness of your treatment and make adjustments as needed.

6. Advocate for Yourself:

Advocate for yourself by speaking up if you feel like your pain is not being adequately managed or if you have concerns about your treatment plan. Don't be afraid to seek a second opinion if needed.

Taking a proactive approach to your care, being honest and open with your healthcare providers, following treatment plans, practicing self-care, tracking your progress, and advocating for yourself can all help you get the best outcomes from your treatment and management of chronic pain.


Diagnosing chronic pain can be a complex and challenging process, as it often involves identifying an underlying cause or condition that is contributing to the pain. Healthcare providers and pain management specialists will typically begin the diagnostic process by conducting a thorough medical history and physical examination, which may involve a range of diagnostic tests, including imaging studies, nerve conduction tests, and blood tests.

One of the key challenges in diagnosing chronic pain is that it can be subjective, with individuals experiencing pain differently and reporting different levels of pain intensity. As such, healthcare providers and pain management specialists may rely on a range of subjective and objective measures to assess and diagnose chronic pain, including self-reported pain scales and clinical assessments.

## Treatment of Chronic Pain

The treatment of chronic pain will depend on the underlying cause of the pain, as well as the severity and duration of the pain. In some cases, pain management may involve a combination of medical interventions, lifestyle modifications, and psychological support.

Medical interventions for chronic pain may include a range of medications, including painkillers, anti-inflammatory drugs, and antidepressants. Physical therapy and alternative therapies such as acupuncture, massage, or chiropractic care may also be recommended to help manage chronic pain.

Lifestyle modifications can also be an effective way to manage chronic pain, particularly in cases where pain is caused or exacerbated by poor lifestyle habits such as smoking, poor diet, or lack of exercise. Adopting healthy habits such as regular exercise, a balanced diet, and stress reduction techniques like meditation or mindfulness can help reduce pain intensity and improve overall well-being.

In addition to medical interventions and lifestyle modifications, psychological support can also be an essential component of chronic pain management. Chronic pain can be emotionally and psychologically challenging, and psychological support, such as counselling or therapy, can help individuals living with chronic pain to develop coping strategies and improve their overall quality of life.

In some cases, surgery may be necessary to treat the underlying cause of chronic pain, particularly in cases where pain is caused by a structural issue, such as a herniated disc or spinal stenosis.

Overall, the treatment of chronic pain will depend on the individual's specific condition and needs. By taking a comprehensive and personalized approach to pain management, healthcare providers and pain management specialists can help individuals living with chronic pain to improve their quality of life and manage their condition more effectively.

Understanding how chronic pain is diagnosed

Diagnosing chronic pain can be a complex and challenging process, as it often involves identifying an underlying cause or condition that is contributing to the pain. Healthcare providers and pain management specialists will typically begin the diagnostic process by conducting a thorough medical history and physical examination, which may involve a range of diagnostic tests, including imaging studies, nerve conduction tests, and blood tests.

One of the key challenges in diagnosing chronic pain is that it can be subjective, with individuals experiencing pain differently and reporting various levels of pain intensity. As such, healthcare providers and pain management specialists may rely on a range of subjective and objective measures to assess and diagnose chronic pain, including self-reported pain scales and clinical assessments.

During the initial medical evaluation, the healthcare provider will typically ask the individual about the location, severity, and duration of their pain, as well as any other symptoms or medical conditions that may be contributing to the pain. The provider will also conduct a physical examination to assess for any visible signs of injury or inflammation.

Diagnostic tests may also be conducted to help identify the underlying cause of chronic pain. Imaging studies, such as X-rays, CT scans, and MRI scans, can help identify structural issues, such as herniated discs or spinal stenosis, which may be contributing to the pain. Nerve conduction tests can help evaluate the function of the nerves and identify any abnormalities that may be causing neuropathic pain.

Blood tests may also be conducted to evaluate for any underlying medical conditions, such as infections or autoimmune disorders, that may be contributing to the pain. In some cases, the healthcare provider may also refer the individual to a specialist, such as a rheumatologist or neurologist, for further evaluation and treatment.

In addition to these diagnostic tests, healthcare providers and pain management specialists may also rely on self-reported pain scales and clinical assessments to help diagnose chronic pain. Self-reported pain scales allow individuals to rate the intensity and duration of their pain, providing a subjective measure of pain severity. Clinical assessments may involve physical tests, such as range of motion tests or muscle strength tests, to help evaluate the underlying cause of the pain.

Diagnosing chronic pain requires a comprehensive and personalized approach, incorporating a range of subjective and objective measures to assess pain severity and identify the underlying cause of the pain. By taking a comprehensive and personalized approach to pain management, healthcare providers and pain management specialists can help individuals living with chronic pain to improve their quality of life and manage their condition more effectively.

Overview of different treatment options, such as medication, physical therapy, and alternative therapies

There are several different treatment options available for managing chronic pain, including medications, physical therapy, and alternative therapies. The choice of treatment will depend on the underlying cause of the pain, as well as the individual's specific needs and preferences.

Medications are a common treatment option for chronic pain and can include a range of drugs, such as painkillers, anti-inflammatory drugs, and antidepressants. Painkillers, such as opioids and nonsteroidal anti-inflammatory drugs (NSAIDs), can help reduce pain intensity and improve quality of life for individuals living with chronic pain. Antidepressants can also be effective in managing chronic pain, particularly in cases where the pain is caused or exacerbated by depression or anxiety.

Physical therapy / physiotherapy is another common treatment option for chronic pain and involves a range of exercises and techniques designed to improve strength, flexibility, and range of motion. Physical therapy can be particularly effective in managing musculoskeletal conditions such as arthritis or back pain. Additionally, physical therapy can help improve overall mobility and function, allowing individuals with chronic pain to participate in activities that they enjoy.

Alternative therapies can also be effective in managing chronic pain, particularly for individuals who may be looking for non-medication-based approaches to pain management. Examples of alternative therapies for chronic pain include:

Acupuncture is a complementary therapy that involves the insertion of thin needles into specific points on the body to stimulate and balance the body's energy flow or Qi. It is a traditional Chinese medicine technique that has been used for thousands of years to manage pain and other health conditions.

Acupuncture is based on the principle that the body has channels or meridians through which Qi flows. When Qi is disrupted or blocked, it can result in pain and other health problems. Acupuncture works by restoring the balance of Qi flow through the stimulation of specific points on the body.

Research has shown that acupuncture can be an effective treatment for chronic pain conditions, including low back pain, neck pain, osteoarthritis, and migraines. It has been suggested that acupuncture may work by stimulating the release of endorphins, which are natural pain-relieving chemicals in the body.

In addition to pain management, acupuncture has been used to treat a variety of health conditions, including anxiety, depression, insomnia, and infertility. Acupuncture is generally considered safe when performed by a licensed and trained practitioner using sterile needles.

While acupuncture may not work for everyone, it can be a useful complementary therapy for managing chronic pain and other health conditions. It is important to discuss any complementary therapies, including acupuncture, with your healthcare provider before beginning treatment. They can help you determine if acupuncture is a safe and appropriate treatment option for your specific condition.

massage therapy

Massage therapy is a complementary therapy that involves the manipulation of soft tissues in the body, including muscles, tendons, and ligaments. It is a manual therapy that can be used to manage pain, reduce stress, and promote relaxation.

Massage therapy involves various techniques, such as Swedish massage, deep tissue massage, and trigger point therapy. These techniques can be applied to different parts of the body, including the back, neck, arms, legs, and feet.

Benefits of Massage Therapy:

1. Pain Management:

Massage therapy can be an effective treatment for managing chronic pain conditions, such as low back pain, neck pain, and osteoarthritis. Massage therapy works by increasing blood flow and oxygen to the affected area, which can help reduce inflammation and promote healing.

Massage therapy can also help reduce muscle tension and stiffness, which can contribute to pain and discomfort. Massage therapy can be particularly useful for individuals with chronic pain who may not be able to tolerate other forms of treatment, such as medication or surgery.

2. Stress Reduction:

Massage therapy can help reduce stress and promote relaxation. Massage therapy works by stimulating the production of endorphins, which are natural mood-boosting chemicals in the body.

Massage therapy can also help reduce the levels of cortisol, a stress hormone, in the body. By reducing stress and promoting relaxation, massage therapy can help improve overall well-being and quality of life.

3. Improved Range of Motion:

Massage therapy can help improve range of motion and flexibility in the body. Massage therapy works by increasing blood flow and oxygen to the muscles, which can help reduce muscle tension and improve mobility.

Massage therapy can also help break up scar tissue and adhesions in the muscles, which can limit movement and cause pain. By improving range of motion and flexibility, massage therapy can help individuals perform daily activities more easily and with less pain.

4. Improved Sleep:

Massage therapy can help improve sleep quality and quantity. Massage therapy works by reducing stress and promoting relaxation, which can help improve sleep.

Massage therapy can also help reduce pain and discomfort, which can interfere with sleep. By improving sleep quality and quantity, massage therapy can help improve overall well-being and quality of life.

Types of Massage Therapy:

1. Swedish Massage:

Swedish massage is a gentle form of massage that involves long strokes, kneading, and circular movements on the superficial layers of muscles. It is a relaxing massage that can help reduce stress and promote relaxation.

2. Deep Tissue Massage:

Deep tissue massage is a more intense form of massage that involves deep pressure and slower movements. It is used to target deeper layers of muscles and can be useful for managing chronic pain conditions.

3. Trigger Point Therapy:

Trigger point therapy involves the application of pressure to specific points in the body that are tender or painful. These points are known as trigger points and can cause pain and discomfort in other areas of the body.

Trigger point therapy can help reduce muscle tension and improve range of motion. It can be useful for managing chronic pain conditions and improving mobility.

Safety Considerations:

Massage therapy is generally considered safe when performed by a trained and licensed practitioner. However, there are some safety considerations to keep in mind.

Massage therapy should be avoided if you have an open wound, skin infection, or a history of blood clots. Massage therapy should also be avoided if you are pregnant or have certain medical conditions, such as osteoporosis or cancer.

It is important to discuss any health conditions or concerns with your healthcare provider before beginning massage therapy. They can help you determine if massage therapy is a safe and appropriate treatment option for you.

Massage therapy is a complementary therapy that can be used to manage pain, reduce stress, and promote relaxation. It can be useful for managing chronic pain conditions, improving range of motion, and promoting overall well-being.

Massage therapy involves various techniques, such as Swedish massage, deep tissue massage, and trigger point therapy, each of which can be tailored to an individual's needs and preferences.

Massage therapy is generally considered safe when performed by a licensed and trained practitioner. However, it is important to discuss any health conditions or concerns with your healthcare provider before beginning massage therapy. They can help you determine if massage therapy is a safe and appropriate treatment option for you.

If you decide to try massage therapy, it is important to find a licensed and trained practitioner who is experienced in the type of massage you are interested in. You should also feel comfortable with the practitioner and communicate any preferences or concerns you may have during the session.

During a massage therapy session, the practitioner will typically ask about your medical history, any pain or discomfort you may be experiencing, and your preferences for the massage. They may also provide suggestions for aftercare, such as drinking water or stretching.

Massage therapy can be an effective complement to other pain management strategies, such as medication and physical therapy. It can also be used as a preventive measure to reduce stress and promote overall well-being.

In conclusion, massage therapy is a complementary therapy that can be used to manage pain, reduce stress, and promote relaxation. It is generally considered safe when performed by a licensed and trained practitioner and can be tailored to an individual's needs and preferences. If you are interested in trying massage therapy, talk to your healthcare provider to determine if it is a safe and appropriate treatment option for you.

Myoskeletal Alignment Therapy,

Myoskeletal Alignment Therapy (MAT) is a form of bodywork developed by Eric Dalton, a renowned manual therapist, and educator. It is a holistic approach that addresses the root cause of pain and dysfunction in the body by restoring proper alignment and movement patterns.

MAT is based on the premise that the body is a complex system of interconnected muscles, bones, and joints that must work together to function properly. When one part of the system is out of alignment, it can lead to pain and dysfunction in other parts of the body.

MAT involves a combination of deep tissue massage, myofascial release, and joint mobilization techniques to restore proper alignment and movement patterns. The therapist works with the client to identify areas of dysfunction and pain, and then applies specific techniques to address these issues.

MAT also incorporates education and self-care strategies to help clients maintain the benefits of the therapy. Clients are taught corrective exercises and self-massage techniques to help them manage their pain and prevent future dysfunction.

MAT can be used to treat a variety of conditions, including low back pain, neck pain, shoulder pain, hip pain, and headaches. It can also be used to improve athletic performance and prevent injuries.

Eric Dalton, the founder of MAT, is a licensed massage therapist and a nationally certified sports massage therapist. He has over 30 years of experience in the manual therapy field and has trained thousands of therapists worldwide in MAT techniques.

MAT has gained popularity in recent years as a holistic approach to pain management and injury prevention. It is often used in conjunction with other therapies, such as physical therapy and chiropractic care, to provide a comprehensive approach to pain management and rehabilitation.

In conclusion, Myoskeletal Alignment Therapy (MAT) is a holistic approach to pain management and injury prevention that addresses the root cause of pain and dysfunction in the body. It is based on the premise that the body is a complex system of interconnected muscles, bones, and joints that must work together to function properly. MAT involves a combination of deep tissue massage, myofascial release, and joint mobilization techniques to restore proper alignment and movement patterns. With the help of a trained MAT practitioner, clients can manage their pain and prevent future dysfunction through education and self-care strategies.

MAT can benefit individuals of all ages and fitness levels, from athletes to those with sedentary lifestyles. It can help improve posture, increase range of motion, and reduce pain and tension in the body.

MAT is typically performed on a massage table with the client fully clothed or draped with a sheet or towel. The therapist may use their hands, fingers, elbows, or other tools to apply pressure to specific areas of the body to release tension and restore proper alignment.

During a MAT session, the therapist will work with the client to identify areas of dysfunction and pain. They may perform a series of assessments and tests to determine the underlying cause of the pain or dysfunction. Based on this information, they will develop a customized treatment plan that may involve a combination of massage techniques, stretching, and corrective exercises.

MAT can be a highly effective form of pain management and injury prevention, but it is important to work with a trained and licensed practitioner who is experienced in the techniques and principles of MAT. They can help identify the underlying cause of pain and dysfunction, and

Following MAT sessions, clients may be provided with home exercises and self-massage techniques to help maintain the benefits of the therapy between sessions. These exercises and techniques can help improve posture, increase mobility, and reduce pain and tension in the body.

Myoskeletal Alignment Therapy (MAT) is a holistic approach to pain management and injury prevention that involves a combination of massage techniques, stretching, and corrective exercises. It can benefit individuals of all ages and fitness levels, and can help improve posture, increase range of motion, and reduce pain and tension in the body. With the help of a trained and licensed practitioner MMT, clients can develop a customized treatment plan to address the underlying cause of pain and dysfunction and maintain the benefits of the therapy over time.

Fascial Therapy,

Fascial therapy is a form of bodywork that focuses on the fascia, a connective tissue that surrounds and supports muscles, bones, and organs in the body. It involves the manipulation of the fascia to release tension, improve mobility, and reduce pain and discomfort in the body.

Fascia is a complex web-like structure that provides support and stability to the body. It is made up of collagen and elastin fibres and is responsible for transmitting forces and movement throughout the body.

When the fascia becomes tight or restricted, it can lead to pain and discomfort in the body. Fascial therapy works by applying pressure to specific areas of the fascia to release tension and improve mobility.

Fascial therapy techniques can include deep tissue massage, myofascial release, and stretching. These techniques can be applied to different parts of the body, including the back, neck, arms, legs, and feet.

Benefits of Fascial Therapy:

1. Pain Management:

Fascial therapy can be an effective treatment for managing chronic pain conditions, such as low back pain, neck pain, and fibromyalgia. Fascial therapy works by releasing tension in the fascia, which can reduce pain and discomfort in the body.

2. Improved Mobility:

Fascial therapy can help improve range of motion and flexibility in the body. It works by releasing tension and restrictions in the fascia, which can improve mobility and movement patterns.

3. Improved Posture:

Fascial therapy can help improve posture by releasing tension and restrictions in the fascia. This can help reduce muscle imbalances and improve alignment in the body.

4. Stress Reduction:

Fascial therapy can help reduce stress and promote relaxation. It works by releasing tension in the fascia, which can help reduce stress and promote relaxation.

Types of Fascial Therapy:

1. Deep Tissue Massage:

Deep tissue massage involves applying pressure to the deep layers of muscle tissue to release tension and reduce pain and discomfort.

2. Myofascial Release:

Myofascial release involves applying gentle pressure to the fascia to release tension and improve mobility. It can be used to treat a variety of conditions, including fibromyalgia and chronic pain.

3. Stretching:

Stretching can be used to release tension and restrictions in the fascia. It can help improve range of motion and flexibility in the body.

Safety Considerations:

Fascial therapy is generally considered safe when performed by a trained and licensed practitioner. However, there are some safety considerations to keep in mind.

Fascial therapy should be avoided if you have an open wound, skin infection, or a history of blood clots. Fascial therapy should also be avoided if you are pregnant or have certain medical conditions, such as osteoporosis or cancer.

It is important to discuss any health conditions or concerns with your healthcare provider before beginning fascial therapy. They can help you determine if fascial therapy is a safe and appropriate treatment option for you.

Fascial therapy is a form of bodywork that focuses on the fascia, a connective tissue that surrounds and supports muscles, bones, and organs in the body. It can be an effective treatment for managing chronic pain conditions, improving mobility, and reducing stress and discomfort in the body.

chiropractic care,

Chiropractic care is a form of complementary and alternative medicine that focuses on the diagnosis, treatment, and prevention of disorders of the musculoskeletal system, particularly the spine. Chiropractors use hands-on techniques, such as spinal manipulation and mobilization, to restore proper alignment and function of the spine and other joints in the body.

The underlying principle of chiropractic care is that the body has an innate ability to heal itself, and that proper alignment of the musculoskeletal system is essential for this healing process to occur. Chiropractors believe that misalignments or subluxations of the spine can interfere with the body's natural healing processes, leading to pain, dysfunction, and other health problems.

Chiropractic care can be used to treat a variety of conditions, including low back pain, neck pain, headaches, and other musculoskeletal disorders. It can also be used to improve overall health and wellness by promoting proper alignment and function of the musculoskeletal system.

Chiropractic techniques can include spinal manipulation, mobilization, and soft tissue therapy. These techniques can be applied to different parts of the body, including the spine, shoulders, hips, and knees.

Benefits of Chiropractic Care:

1. Pain Management:

Chiropractic care can be an effective treatment for managing pain and discomfort in the body. Chiropractors use hands-on techniques to restore proper alignment and function of the musculoskeletal system, which can reduce pain and improve mobility.

2. Improved Mobility:

Chiropractic care can help improve range of motion and flexibility in the body. It works by restoring proper alignment and function of the musculoskeletal system, which can improve movement patterns and reduce muscle imbalances.

3. Improved Posture:

Chiropractic care can help improve posture by restoring proper alignment and function of the spine and other joints in the body. This can help reduce muscle imbalances and improve alignment in the body.

4. Improved Overall Health:

Chiropractic care can help improve overall health and wellness by promoting proper alignment and function of the musculoskeletal system. It can also help reduce stress and promote relaxation, which can have a positive impact on overall health and well-being.

Safety Considerations:

Chiropractic care is generally considered safe when performed by a trained and licensed chiropractor. However, there are some safety considerations to keep in mind.

Chiropractic care should be avoided if you have certain medical conditions, such as osteoporosis or cancer. It should also be avoided if you have an increased risk of stroke or certain spinal conditions.

It is important to discuss any health conditions or concerns with your healthcare provider before beginning chiropractic care. They can help you determine if chiropractic care is a safe and appropriate treatment option for you.

Osteopathic Care

Osteopathic care is a form of complementary and alternative medicine that focuses on the diagnosis, treatment, and prevention of disorders of the musculoskeletal system, particularly the spine. Osteopaths use hands-on techniques, such as spinal manipulation, soft tissue therapy, and joint mobilization, to restore proper alignment and function of the body.

The underlying principle of osteopathic care is that the body has an innate ability to heal itself, and that proper alignment of the musculoskeletal system is essential for this healing process to occur. Osteopaths believe that misalignments or restrictions of the spine and other joints can interfere with the body's natural healing processes, leading to pain, dysfunction, and other health problems.

Osteopathic care can be used to treat a variety of conditions, including low back pain, neck pain, headaches, and other musculoskeletal disorders. It can also be used to improve overall health and wellness by promoting proper alignment and function of the body.

Osteopathic techniques can include spinal manipulation, soft tissue therapy, joint mobilization, and other hands-on techniques. These techniques can be applied to different parts of the body, including the spine, shoulders, hips, and knees.

Benefits of Osteopathic Care:

1. Pain Management:

Osteopathic care can be an effective treatment for managing pain and discomfort in the body. Osteopaths use hands-on techniques to restore proper alignment and function of the musculoskeletal system, which can reduce pain and improve mobility.

2. Improved Mobility:

Osteopathic care can help improve range of motion and flexibility in the body. It works by restoring proper alignment and function of the musculoskeletal system, which can improve movement patterns and reduce muscle imbalances.

3. Improved Posture:

Osteopathic care can help improve posture by restoring proper alignment and function of the spine and other joints in the body. This can help reduce muscle imbalances and improve alignment in the body.

4. Improved Overall Health:

Osteopathic care can help improve overall health and wellness by promoting proper alignment and function of the musculoskeletal system. It can also help reduce stress and promote relaxation, which can have a positive impact on overall health and well-being.

Safety Considerations:

Osteopathic care is generally considered safe when performed by a trained and licensed osteopath. However, there are some safety considerations to keep in mind.

Osteopathic care should be avoided if you have certain medical conditions, such as osteoporosis or cancer. It should also be avoided if you have an increased risk of stroke or certain spinal conditions.

It is important to discuss any health conditions or concerns with your healthcare provider before beginning osteopathic care. They can help you determine if osteopathic care is a safe and appropriate treatment option

Osteopathic care is a form of complementary and alternative medicine that focuses on the diagnosis, treatment, and prevention of disorders of the musculoskeletal system, particularly the spine. It can be an effective treatment for managing pain and discomfort in the body, improving mobility and posture, and promoting overall health and wellness.

Yoga

Yoga is a mind-body practice that originated in ancient India and has become increasingly popular in the West over the past few decades. It involves a combination of physical postures, breathing exercises, meditation, and relaxation techniques to promote overall health and well-being.

The physical postures, or asanas, in yoga are designed to stretch and strengthen the body, improve flexibility and balance, and promote relaxation. They range from gentle, restorative poses to more challenging, advanced poses that require strength and balance.

In addition to the physical benefits, yoga has been shown to have a positive impact on mental health. The breathing exercises and meditation techniques in yoga can help reduce stress and anxiety, improve concentration, focus, and promote a sense of calm and well-being.

Benefits of Yoga:

1. Improved Flexibility:

Yoga can help improve flexibility by stretching and lengthening the muscles and connective tissues in the body. Regular yoga practice can help increase range of motion and prevent injuries.

2. Increased Strength:

Yoga can help increase strength by using the body's own weight to build muscle. The physical postures in yoga can target specific muscle groups, helping to improve overall strength and endurance.

3. Stress Reduction:

Yoga can help reduce stress and promote relaxation by incorporating breathing exercises and meditation techniques. These practices can help calm the mind and reduce anxiety, leading to a greater sense of well-being.

4. Improved Posture:

Yoga can help improve posture by strengthening the muscles that support the spine and promoting proper alignment of the body. This can help reduce pain and discomfort in the body.

5. Improved Overall Health:

Yoga can help improve overall health by reducing stress, improving flexibility and strength, and promoting relaxation. It has also been shown to have a positive impact on other health conditions, such as cardiovascular disease, diabetes, and chronic pain.

Types of Yoga:

There are many different types of yoga, each with its own unique focus and approach. Some of the most common types of yoga include:

1. Hatha Yoga:

Hatha yoga is a gentle, slow-paced form of yoga that focuses on the physical postures and breathing exercises.

2. Vinyasa Yoga:

Vinyasa yoga is a more dynamic, flowing form of yoga that emphasizes movement and breath coordination.

3. Ashtanga Yoga:

Ashtanga yoga is a physically challenging form of yoga that involves a series of set postures performed in a specific sequence.

4. Restorative Yoga:

Restorative yoga is a gentle, relaxing form of yoga that involves supported poses designed to promote deep relaxation and stress relief.

Safety Considerations:

Yoga is generally considered safe for most people, but it is important to practice with awareness and caution. It is important to listen to your body and avoid pushing beyond your limits.

If you have any health concerns or medical conditions, it is important to speak with your healthcare provider before beginning a yoga practice. They can help you determine if yoga is safe and appropriate for you and can provide guidance on modifications or adjustments to make to your practice.

Pilates

Pilates is a form of exercise that was developed in the early 20th century by Joseph Pilates. It is a mind-body practice that emphasizes proper alignment, core strength, and flexibility.

The exercises in Pilates focus on controlled movements and proper breathing techniques. They are designed to improve posture, balance, and overall strength and flexibility. Pilates can be done using a mat or with specialized equipment, such as the reformer.

Benefits of Pilates:

1. Improved Core Strength:

Pilates can help improve core strength by targeting the deep abdominal muscles, as well as the muscles of the back, hips, and pelvis. Strong core muscles can help improve posture, reduce back pain, and improve overall physical function.

2. Improved Flexibility:

Pilates can help improve flexibility by stretching and lengthening the muscles in the body. The controlled movements and breathing techniques in Pilates can help improve range of motion and prevent injuries.

3. Improved Posture:

Pilates can help improve posture by strengthening the muscles that support the spine and promoting proper alignment of the body. This can help reduce pain and discomfort in the body.

4. Stress Reduction:

Pilates can help reduce stress and promote relaxation by incorporating breathing exercises and meditation techniques. These practices can help calm the mind and reduce anxiety, leading to a greater sense of well-being.

Types of Pilates:

There are two main types of Pilates:

1. Mat Pilates:

Mat Pilates involves a series of exercises done on a mat, using only body weight for resistance.

2. Equipment-Based Pilates:

Equipment-based Pilates involves the use of specialized equipment, such as the reformer, to add resistance and support to the exercises.

Safety Considerations:

Pilates is generally considered safe for most people, but it is important to practice with awareness and caution. It is important to listen to your body and avoid pushing beyond your limits.

If you have any health concerns or medical conditions, it is important to speak with your healthcare provider before beginning a Pilates practice. They can help you determine if Pilates is safe and appropriate for you and can provide guidance on modifications or adjustments to make to your practice.

These therapies may help reduce pain intensity, improve overall well-being, and promote relaxation and stress reduction.

In some cases, surgery may be necessary to treat the underlying cause of chronic pain, particularly in cases where pain is caused by a structural issue, such as a herniated disc or spinal stenosis.

It is important to note that not all treatments will be effective for every individual with chronic pain. It may be necessary to try several different treatments or combinations of treatments to find the most effective approach to pain management. Additionally, healthcare providers and pain management specialists may work with individuals to develop a comprehensive pain management plan that incorporates several different approaches to managing chronic pain.

Overall, there are several different treatment options available for managing chronic pain, including medications, physical therapy, alternative therapies, and surgery. By working with healthcare providers and pain management specialists, individuals with chronic pain can develop a personalized treatment plan that addresses their specific needs and preferences and improves their quality of life.

Explanation of how to work with healthcare providers to create a personalized treatment plan

Working with healthcare providers is an essential component of developing a personalized treatment plan for chronic pain. Effective communication and collaboration with healthcare providers can help individuals living with chronic pain to identify the most appropriate treatment options and improve their overall quality of life.

One of the first steps in working with healthcare providers is to establish a relationship of trust and open communication. It is essential to be honest and open about your pain symptoms, concerns, and preferences. This will help the healthcare provider to understand your specific needs and develop a personalized treatment plan that is tailored to your unique situation.

During the initial consultation, the healthcare provider will typically conduct a thorough medical history and physical examination and may also conduct diagnostic tests to help identify the underlying cause of the pain. Based on this information, the healthcare provider will work with you to develop a personalized treatment plan that addresses your specific needs and preferences.

In developing a personalized treatment plan, the healthcare provider may recommend a range of treatment options, including medications, physical therapy, and alternative therapies. It is important to ask questions and clarify any concerns or uncertainties about the recommended treatments to ensure that you have a clear understanding of the benefits and risks associated with each treatment option.

Additionally, it is important to be an active participant in your treatment plan by following the recommended treatment regimen and keeping the healthcare provider informed of any changes or improvements in your symptoms. Regular follow-up appointments and ongoing communication with the healthcare provider are essential for evaluating the effectiveness of the treatment plan and making adjustments as needed.

In addition to working with the healthcare provider, it may also be helpful to seek support from other resources, such as pain management specialists, physical therapists, and mental health professionals. These resources can provide additional guidance and support in managing chronic pain and developing effective coping strategies.

Overall, working with healthcare providers is essential for developing a personalized treatment plan for chronic pain. By establishing a relationship of trust and open communication, individuals with chronic pain can work with their healthcare providers to identify the most appropriate treatment options and improve their overall quality of life.

Strategies for finding and working with a pain management team

Living with chronic pain can be challenging, and finding a pain management team that you trust and feel comfortable working with is essential for effective pain management. Here are some strategies for finding and working with a pain management team:

1. Ask for referrals: Ask your primary care physician for a referral to a pain management specialist or a pain management clinic. You can also ask friends or family members for recommendations.
2. Do your research: Once you have a list of potential pain management teams, do some research to learn more about them. Look up their credentials, experience, and patient reviews. This can help you narrow down your options and choose a pain management team that is best suited to your needs.
3. Schedule a consultation: Schedule a consultation with the pain management team to discuss your pain symptoms, medical history, and treatment options. This can give you a sense of their approach

to pain management and help you determine whether they are a good fit for you.

4. Communicate openly: Effective communication is essential for developing a personalized treatment plan for chronic pain. Be open and honest about your pain symptoms, concerns, and preferences. Ask questions and clarify any uncertainties you may have about the recommended treatment options.

5. Participate actively: Be an active participant in your treatment plan by following the recommended treatment regimen and keeping the pain management team informed of any changes or improvements in your symptoms. Regular follow-up appointments and ongoing communication with the pain management team are essential for evaluating the effectiveness of the treatment plan and making adjustments as needed.

6. Seek support: In addition to working with the pain management team, it may also be helpful to seek support from other resources, such as physical therapists, mental health professionals, and support groups. These resources can provide additional guidance and support in managing chronic pain and developing effective coping strategies.

Overall, finding and working with a pain management team that you trust and feel comfortable with is essential for effective pain management. By following these strategies, individuals with chronic pain can identify the most appropriate treatment options and develop a personalized treatment plan that addresses their specific needs and preferences.

# Chapter 3

## The Role of Lifestyle Changes in Managing Chronic Pain

### Overview of Lifestyle Changes for Chronic Pain Management

Lifestyle changes can play a critical role in managing chronic pain. By adopting healthy habits, individuals with chronic pain can improve their overall well-being, reduce pain intensity, and increase their ability to perform daily activities.

One of the key lifestyle changes for chronic pain management is regular exercise. Exercise can help improve flexibility, strength, and range of motion, and can also help reduce pain intensity. Low-impact exercises such as walking, swimming, and yoga are particularly effective for managing chronic pain.

Dietary changes can also be effective in managing chronic pain. A diet that is high in anti-inflammatory foods, such as fruits, vegetables, and omega-3 fatty acids, can help reduce inflammation and pain intensity.

Additionally, reducing or eliminating foods that are high in sugar, caffeine, and processed foods can help reduce pain intensity.

Stress reduction techniques, such as meditation, mindfulness, and deep breathing, can also be effective in managing chronic pain. Stress can exacerbate pain symptoms, and learning effective stress management techniques can help reduce pain intensity and improve overall well-being.

## Implementing Lifestyle Changes for Chronic Pain Management

Implementing lifestyle changes for chronic pain management can be challenging, particularly for individuals who may be experiencing limited mobility or difficulty performing daily activities. However, making small, gradual changes over time can help individuals with chronic pain to adopt healthy habits and improve their quality of life.

One effective approach to implementing lifestyle changes for chronic pain management is to work with a healthcare provider or pain management specialist to develop a comprehensive pain management plan that incorporates lifestyle changes, such as exercise and dietary modifications.

Additionally, seeking support from friends, family members, and support groups can be helpful in adopting and maintaining healthy lifestyle habits. Accountability partners can help individuals with chronic pain to stay motivated and committed to their goals.

It is also important to set realistic goals and to make changes gradually over time. Adopting too many lifestyle changes at once can be overwhelming and may lead to frustration and burnout.

Overall, lifestyle changes can play a critical role in managing chronic pain. By adopting healthy habits, individuals with chronic pain can reduce pain intensity, improve their overall well-being, and increase their ability to perform daily activities. By working with healthcare providers, seeking support from others, and making changes gradually over time, individuals with chronic pain can implement lifestyle changes effectively and improve their quality of life.

Explanation of how lifestyle changes can affect chronic pain
Lifestyle changes can have a significant impact on chronic pain, as they can help improve overall health and reduce pain intensity. By adopting healthy habits, individuals with chronic pain can improve their physical, mental, and emotional well-being, which can help reduce pain symptoms and improve overall quality of life.

Exercise is one lifestyle change that can have a significant impact on chronic pain. Regular exercise can help improve flexibility, strength, and range of motion, which can help reduce pain intensity and improve overall function. Additionally, exercise can help release endorphins, which are natural painkillers that can help reduce pain intensity and improve mood.

Dietary changes can also be effective in managing chronic pain. A diet that is high in anti-inflammatory foods, such as fruits, vegetables, and omega-3 fatty acids, can help reduce inflammation and pain intensity. Additionally, reducing or eliminating foods that are high in sugar, caffeine, and processed foods can help reduce pain symptoms.

Stress reduction techniques, such as meditation, mindfulness, and deep breathing, can also be effective in managing chronic pain. Stress can exacerbate pain symptoms, and learning effective stress management techniques can help reduce pain intensity and improve overall well-being.

Sleep hygiene is another important lifestyle change that can affect chronic pain. Getting adequate sleep is essential for overall health and can help reduce pain intensity. Additionally, creating a relaxing sleep environment, such as a cool and dark room, can help promote restful sleep.

Overall, lifestyle changes can have a significant impact on chronic pain. By adopting healthy habits, individuals with chronic pain can improve their overall well-being, reduce pain intensity, and increase their ability to perform daily activities. By working with healthcare providers and making changes gradually over time, individuals with chronic pain can implement lifestyle changes effectively and improve their quality of life.

Tips for creating a supportive and safe environment for rehabilitation Strategies for Adopting Healthy Habits:

1. Set realistic goals: Start small and work your way up. Set achievable goals, such as exercising for 15 minutes a day or adding one serving of fruits or vegetables to your daily diet.
2. Create a plan: Develop a plan for adopting healthy habits. This could include scheduling exercise time, planning meals, and setting aside time for relaxation and stress reduction.
3. Find support: Seek support from friends, family members, or a support group. An accountability partner can help keep you motivated and on track.
4. Gradually make changes: Make changes gradually over time. Trying to change everything at once can be overwhelming and may lead to burnout.
5. Monitor progress: Keep track of progress towards your goals. This can help you stay motivated and make adjustments as needed.

Tips for Creating a Supportive and Safe Environment for Rehabilitation:

1. Consult with healthcare providers: Work with healthcare providers to develop a rehabilitation plan that is safe and appropriate for your specific needs.
2. Set up a safe space: Create a safe and supportive environment for rehabilitation by removing any potential hazards or obstacles, such as loose rugs or clutter.
3. Use appropriate equipment: Use appropriate equipment for exercise or rehabilitation, such as supportive shoes, a comfortable exercise mat, or resistance bands.

4. Work with a physical therapist: Consider working with a physical therapist who can help guide you through exercises and ensure proper form to reduce the risk of injury.
5. Seek support: Seek support from friends, family members, or a support group. Having a support system can help you stay motivated and committed to your rehabilitation goals.

Overall, adopting healthy habits such as nutrition, exercise, and sleep, and creating a supportive and safe environment for rehabilitation are essential components of managing chronic pain. By following these strategies, individuals with chronic pain can improve their overall well-being, reduce pain intensity, and improve their quality of life.

Strategies for adopting healthy habits such as nutrition, exercise, and sleep

Adopting healthy habits such as nutrition, exercise, and sleep is essential for managing chronic pain. Here are some strategies for adopting healthy habits:

1. Start small: Start with small, achievable goals. For example, you could aim to eat one extra serving of vegetables each day, walk for 10 minutes a day, or go to bed 15 minutes earlier.
2. Create a plan: Develop a plan for adopting healthy habits. This could include scheduling exercise time, planning meals, and setting aside time for relaxation and stress reduction.

3. Seek support: Seek support from friends, family members, or a support group. An accountability partner can help keep you motivated and on track.
4. Make it enjoyable: Choose activities that you enjoy, such as swimming, dancing, or gardening. This can make it easier to stick to your healthy habits.
5. Monitor progress: Keep track of progress towards your goals. This can help you stay motivated and make adjustments as needed.
6. Focus on balance: Focus on balanced nutrition, including plenty of fruits, vegetables, whole grains, lean proteins, and healthy fats. Aim for at least 150 minutes of moderate-intensity exercise per week and try to get 7-9 hours of sleep each night.
7. Be consistent: Consistency is key when adopting healthy habits. Try to incorporate healthy habits into your daily routine and stick to them as much as possible.

Overall, adopting healthy habits such as nutrition, exercise, and sleep is essential for managing chronic pain. By following these strategies, individuals with chronic pain can improve their overall well-being, reduce pain intensity, and improve their quality of life.

Tips for creating a supportive and safe environment for rehabilitation
Creating a supportive and safe environment for rehabilitation is important for individuals with chronic pain. Here are some tips for creating such an environment:

1. Consult with healthcare providers: Work with healthcare providers, such as physical therapists, to develop a rehabilitation plan that is safe and appropriate for your specific needs.
2. Set up a safe space: Create a safe and supportive environment for rehabilitation by removing any potential hazards or obstacles, such as loose rugs or clutter.
3. Use appropriate equipment: Use appropriate equipment for exercise or rehabilitation, such as supportive shoes, a comfortable exercise mat, or resistance bands.
4. Start with low-impact exercises: Begin with low-impact exercises, such as walking or swimming, and gradually increase intensity and duration as your body adjusts.

Here is a sample walking program that can be completed in 40 minutes while keeping your heart rate between 105 and 115 bpm:

- Warm-up (5 minutes): Start with a slow, easy pace for the first 5 minutes to warm up your muscles and gradually increase your heart rate.
- Moderate intensity walk (25 minutes): Aim for a brisk walk that keeps your heart rate between 105 and 115 bpm for 25 minutes. This can be done by walking at a faster pace, increasing the incline or resistance, or incorporating interval training (alternating periods of higher and lower intensity).

- Cool-down (5 minutes): End with a slower pace for the last 5 minutes to cool down your body and gradually lower your heart rate.

- Here are some additional tips to help you achieve your heart rate goals during your walk:

- Use a heart rate monitor or fitness tracker to track your heart rate and adjust your pace as needed.
- Check your breathing rate during the walk. If you are having difficulty breathing or talking, slow down your pace.
- Focus on good posture and proper form to optimize your walking efficiency and reduce the risk of injury.
- Try to incorporate hills or stairs into your walk to increase the intensity and challenge your body.

- Remember, it's important to listen to your body and adjust your walking program as needed to avoid overexertion or injury. By following a consistent walking program and gradually increasing the duration and intensity of your walks, you can improve your cardiovascular health, endurance, and overall well-being.

Also while we are on the subject of exercise here's a sample rehab workout on a:

Recumbent bike

Warm-up: Start with 5-10 minutes of light cycling at a low resistance level to warm up the muscles.

Main Workout:

Interval Training:

- 5 minutes at a moderate pace and resistance level.
- 1 minute at a high pace and resistance level.
- 2 minutes at a low pace and resistance level.
- Repeat the above interval for 20-30 minutes.

Resistance Training:
- 10 minutes of steady-state cycling at a moderate pace and high resistance level.
- 1 minute of easy cycling to recover.
- Repeat the above interval for 20-30 minutes.

Hill Climbing:
- 5 minutes at a moderate pace and low resistance level.
- 5 minutes at a moderate pace and high resistance level.
- 5 minutes at a moderate pace and low resistance level.
- Repeat the above interval for 20-30 minutes.

Cool-down: End with 5-10 minutes of light cycling at a low resistance level to cool down and allow the muscles to recover.

Note: The duration and intensity of the intervals can be adjusted based on the individual's fitness level and rehab goals. It's important to consult with a healthcare professional or physical therapist before beginning any new exercise program, especially if you're recovering from an injury or surgery.

5. Work with a physical therapist: Consider working with a physical therapist who can help guide you through exercises and ensure proper form to reduce the risk of injury.
6. Take breaks: Take breaks as needed during exercise or rehabilitation to avoid overexertion and fatigue.
7. Seek support: Seek support from friends, family members, or a support group. Having a support system can help you stay motivated and committed to your rehabilitation goals.

There are several chronic pain support groups in Australia that can provide resources, information, and community for individuals living with chronic pain. Here are a few options:

- Chronic Pain Australia: This is a national organization that advocates for individuals living with chronic pain and provides resources and support through their website and social media channels. They also have a directory of chronic pain support groups throughout Australia.

- Pain Support ACT: This is a community-based organization that provides support and information for individuals living with chronic pain in the Australian Capital Territory (ACT). They offer peer support groups, information sessions, and advocacy services.
- Pain Management Network: This is a free online support group for individuals living with chronic pain in Australia. The group is moderated by healthcare professionals and offers a forum for members to connect, share experiences, and provide support to one another.
- Chronic Pain Queensland: This is a non-profit organization that provides support and advocacy for individuals living with chronic pain in Queensland. They offer support groups, information sessions, and a directory of healthcare professionals who specialize in chronic pain management.
- PainWISE: This is a multidisciplinary pain management clinic that offers support and resources for individuals living with chronic pain in New South Wales. They provide support groups, educational programs, and access to pain management specialists.

These are just a few examples of chronic pain support groups in Australia. It's important to find a support group that meets your specific needs and interests. You can search online or speak with your healthcare provider for recommendations.

There are many chronic pain support groups in the United States that can provide resources, information, and community for individuals living with chronic pain. Here are a few options:

- American Chronic Pain Association: This is a non-profit organization that provides resources and support for individuals living with chronic pain, as well as their families and healthcare providers. They offer educational materials, support groups, and advocacy services.
- US Pain Foundation: This is a non-profit organization that provides support, education, and advocacy for individuals living with chronic pain. They offer a variety of programs, including support groups, educational webinars, and advocacy initiatives.
- National Fibromyalgia & Chronic Pain Association: This is a non-profit organization that provides resources and support for individuals living with fibromyalgia and other chronic pain conditions. They offer support groups, educational resources, and advocacy services.
- Chronic Pain Anonymous: This is a 12-step program for individuals living with chronic pain who are seeking support and recovery. They offer meetings, resources, and support for individuals who are struggling with chronic pain.
- Pain Connection: This is a non-profit organization that provides support and resources for individuals living with chronic pain. They

offer support groups, educational programs, and advocacy services.

- These are just a few examples of chronic pain support groups in the United States. It's important to find a support group that meets your specific needs and interests. You can search online or speak with your healthcare provider for recommendations.

Europe
- There are many chronic pain support groups in Europe that can provide resources, information, and community for individuals living with chronic pain. Here are a few options:

- European Pain Federation: This is a non-profit organization that provides resources and support for individuals living with chronic pain in Europe. They offer educational materials, support groups, and advocacy services.
- Pain Alliance Europe: This is a non-profit organization that provides support, education, and advocacy for individuals living with chronic pain in Europe. They offer a variety of programs, including support groups, educational resources, and advocacy initiatives.
- Chronic Pain Ireland: This is a non-profit organization that provides support and resources for individuals living with chronic pain in Ireland. They offer support groups, educational resources, and advocacy services.

- Fibromyalgia Association UK: This is a non-profit organization that provides resources and support for individuals living with fibromyalgia and other chronic pain conditions in the United Kingdom. They offer support groups, educational resources, and advocacy services.
- Association Française de la Fibromyalgia: This is a non-profit organization that provides support and resources for individuals living with fibromyalgia and other chronic pain conditions in France. They offer support groups, educational resources, and advocacy services.

- These are just a few examples of chronic pain support groups in Europe. It's important to find a support group that meets your specific needs and interests. You can search online or speak with your healthcare provider for recommendations.

Asia

There are many chronic pain support groups in Asia that can provide resources, information, and community for individuals living with chronic pain. Here are a few options:

- Chronic Pain Association of Singapore: This is a non-profit organization that provides resources and support for individuals living with chronic pain in Singapore. They offer support groups, educational resources, and advocacy services.

- Japan Chronic Pain Association: This is a non-profit organization that provides support and resources for individuals living with chronic pain in Japan. They offer support groups, educational resources, and advocacy services.
- Hong Kong Pain Society: This is a non-profit organization that provides support and resources for individuals living with chronic pain in Hong Kong. They offer support groups, educational resources, and advocacy services.
- Indian Society for Study of Pain: This is a non-profit organization that provides support and resources for individuals living with chronic pain in India. They offer support groups, educational resources, and advocacy services.
- Chronic Pain Malaysia: This is a non-profit organization that provides support and resources for individuals living with chronic pain in Malaysia. They offer support groups, educational resources, and advocacy services.

These are just a few examples of chronic pain support groups in Asia. It's important to find a support group that meets your specific needs and interests. You can search online or speak with your healthcare provider for recommendations.

8. Practice relaxation techniques: Incorporate relaxation techniques, such as deep breathing, meditation, or yoga, into your rehabilitation routine to help manage stress and improve overall well-being.

Overall, creating a supportive and safe environment for rehabilitation is essential for managing chronic pain. By following these tips, individuals with chronic pain can improve their physical function, reduce pain intensity, and improve their overall quality of life.

Ways to integrate relaxation techniques into daily life
Integrating relaxation techniques into daily life can be an effective way to manage chronic pain and improve overall well-being. Here are some ways to incorporate relaxation techniques into your daily routine:

1. Take breaks: Take short breaks throughout the day to practice relaxation techniques, such as deep breathing, mindfulness, or progressive muscle relaxation. Even just a few minutes of relaxation can help reduce stress and tension.
2. Practice yoga or stretching: Incorporate yoga or stretching exercises into your daily routine. These activities can help improve flexibility and range of motion, as well as promote relaxation and stress reduction.
3. Listen to calming music: Listen to calming music, such as classical music or nature sounds, to promote relaxation and reduce stress. Listening to music has been shown to have a positive impact on chronic pain in several ways. Here are a few potential benefits:

- Distraction: Listening to music can help distract the brain from focusing on the pain, which can help reduce the intensity of the pain experience.
- Mood enhancement: Music can improve mood by releasing endorphins and other feel-good chemicals in the brain, which can help individuals with chronic pain feel more positive and relaxed.
- Relaxation: Slow, calming music can help induce a state of relaxation and reduce muscle tension, which can help alleviate pain.
- Brain activity: Music has been shown to activate areas of the brain that are associated with pain modulation, which can help reduce pain sensitivity.
- Memory association: Listening to music that is associated with positive memories can help individuals with chronic pain feel more connected to positive experiences, which can help improve mood and reduce pain.

- While listening to music is not a cure for chronic pain, it can be a helpful adjunctive therapy to help manage symptoms and improve quality of life. It's important to choose music that is calming and enjoyable, and to listen to it in a quiet, comfortable environment.

4. Use guided meditation or visualization: Use guided meditation or visualization exercises to help relax the mind and reduce stress.

There are many apps and resources available that provide guided meditation exercises.
5. Engage in creative activities: Engage in creative activities, such as drawing, painting, or writing, to promote relaxation and reduce stress.
6. Spend time in nature: Spending time in nature, such as going for a walk or spending time in a park, can help promote relaxation and reduce stress. Being in nature has been shown to have a positive impact on chronic pain in several ways. Here are a few potential benefits:

- Stress reduction: Being in nature can help reduce stress, which is a common contributor to chronic pain. Stress reduction techniques such as mindfulness meditation and deep breathing can help alleviate pain and improve overall well-being.
- Sensory distraction: Being in nature provides a sensory-rich environment that can help distract the brain from focusing on pain. The sights, sounds, and smells of nature can help promote relaxation and reduce pain sensitivity.
- Physical activity: Many outdoor activities such as hiking and swimming can help promote physical activity, which can help improve cardiovascular health and reduce pain sensitivity.
- Vitamin D: Exposure to sunlight can help increase levels of vitamin D, which is important for maintaining bone health and reducing inflammation in the body.

- Social connection: Being in nature can provide opportunities for social connection, which is important for maintaining a sense of purpose and well-being. Social support has been shown to have a positive impact on pain management.

- While being in nature is not a cure for chronic pain, it can be a helpful adjunctive therapy to help manage symptoms and improve quality of life. It's important to choose activities that are enjoyable and manageable based on individual abilities and limitations. It's also important to take precautions to avoid overexertion and sun exposure, and to consult with a healthcare provider before starting a new physical activity program.

7. Get enough sleep: Make sure to get enough sleep each night, as adequate sleep is essential for overall well-being and can help reduce stress and tension.

Overall, integrating relaxation techniques into daily life can be an effective way to manage chronic pain and improve overall well-being. By incorporating these practices into your daily routine, you can help promote relaxation, reduce stress, and improve your quality of life.

# Chapter 4

Mind-Body Techniques for Managing Chronic Pain

Mind-body techniques such as mindfulness, meditation, and cognitive-behavioural therapy can be effective in managing chronic pain. Here is an overview of each technique:

1. Mindfulness: Mindfulness involves paying attention to the present moment without judgment. It can help individuals with chronic pain to reduce stress, improve their ability to cope with pain, and increase their overall sense of well-being. Mindfulness techniques can include meditation, breathing exercises, and body scans.
2. Meditation: Meditation involves focusing the mind on a particular object or thought, such as the breath or a sound. It can help individuals with chronic pain to reduce stress, increase relaxation, and improve their ability to cope with pain. Meditation can be practiced in a variety of ways, such as sitting, walking, or even lying down.

Overview of mind-body techniques such as mindfulness, meditation, and cognitive-behavioural therapy

Mind-body techniques are a group of practices that aim to improve physical and mental health by connecting the mind and body. These techniques can be effective in managing chronic pain. Here is an overview of some of the most commonly used mind-body techniques:

1. Mindfulness: Mindfulness involves paying attention to the present moment without judgment. It can help individuals with chronic pain to reduce stress, improve their ability to cope with pain, and increase their overall sense of well-being. Mindfulness techniques can include meditation, breathing exercises, and body scans.
2. Meditation: Meditation involves focusing the mind on a particular object or thought, such as the breath or a sound. It can help individuals with chronic pain to reduce stress, increase relaxation, and improve their ability to cope with pain. Meditation can be practiced in a variety of ways, such as sitting, walking, or even lying down.
- Cognitive-behavioural therapy (CBT): CBT is a type of talk therapy that focuses on changing negative thought patterns and behaviours. It can help individuals with chronic pain to improve their coping skills, reduce pain intensity, and improve their overall quality of life. CBT can include techniques such as relaxation training, cognitive restructuring, and behaviour modification. Cognitive-behavioural therapy (CBT): CBT is a type of talk therapy that

focuses on changing negative thought patterns and behaviours. It can help individuals with chronic pain to improve their coping skills, reduce pain intensity, and improve their overall quality of life. CBT can include techniques such as relaxation training, cognitive restructuring, and behaviour modification. CBT (Cognitive Behavioral Therapy) is a form of psychotherapy that aims to help individuals change negative or unhealthy thought patterns and behaviours that contribute to mental health conditions and other challenges, including chronic pain. Here are a few ways that CBT can benefit individuals:

- Identifies negative thinking patterns: CBT helps individuals recognize negative thinking patterns, such as catastrophizing or negative self-talk, that can contribute to chronic pain and other mental health conditions. By identifying these patterns, individuals can learn to challenge them and replace them with more positive and helpful thoughts.
- Changes behaviour: CBT can help individuals identify and change behaviours that may be contributing to chronic pain, such as avoiding activities or social situations due to fear of pain. By gradually increasing activity levels and exposure to feared situations, individuals can learn to manage their pain more effectively.
- Increases coping skills: CBT can teach individuals coping skills and techniques for managing pain, such as relaxation techniques,

breathing exercises, and mindfulness meditation. These skills can help individuals manage pain symptoms more effectively and improve overall quality of life.
- Promotes problem-solving skills: CBT can help individuals develop problem-solving skills and strategies for addressing challenges related to chronic pain, such as communicating with healthcare providers, managing medication regimens, and setting realistic goals.
- Improves overall mental health: CBT can help individuals manage symptoms of depression, anxiety, and other mental health conditions that may be associated with chronic pain. By improving overall mental health, individuals may experience a reduction in pain symptoms and improved quality of life.

- While CBT is not a cure for chronic pain, it can be a helpful adjunctive therapy to help individuals manage symptoms and improve overall quality of life. It's important to find a qualified and experienced therapist who specializes in CBT and chronic pain management.
3. Overall, mind-body techniques can be effective in managing chronic pain. By incorporating mindfulness, meditation, and cognitive-behavioural therapy techniques into their daily routine, individuals with chronic pain can reduce stress, improve their ability to cope with pain, and improve their overall well-being. It is important to work with a healthcare provider or pain management

specialist to determine which techniques may be most effective for individual needs.

Yoga: Yoga is a mind-body practice that combines physical postures, breathing techniques, and meditation. It can help individuals with chronic pain to improve their flexibility, strength, and balance, as well as reduce stress and tension.

3. Tai chi is a mind-body practice that involves gentle movements, deep breathing, and meditation. It can help individuals with chronic pain to improve their balance, flexibility, and coordination, as well as reduce stress and tension. Tai chi is a traditional Chinese mind-body exercise that involves a series of slow, gentle movements and postures. It has been shown to have several benefits for individuals with chronic pain. Here are a few potential benefits:

- Reduced pain and stiffness: Tai chi can help improve flexibility and reduce stiffness in the joints, which can help alleviate chronic pain symptoms.
- Improved balance: Tai chi can help improve balance and coordination, which can help reduce the risk of falls and other injuries, particularly in older adults.
- Stress reduction: Tai chi can help reduce stress and anxiety, which are common contributors to chronic pain.

- Improved overall fitness: Tai chi can help improve cardiovascular fitness, muscle strength, and flexibility, which can help improve overall physical function and reduce pain symptoms.
- Mindfulness: Tai chi involves a focus on breath and body awareness, which can help individuals become more mindful and present in the moment. This can help reduce stress and improve overall well-being.

- While tai chi is not a cure for chronic pain, it can be a helpful adjunctive therapy to help manage symptoms and improve overall quality of life. It's important to find a qualified instructor who specializes in tai chi and chronic pain management, and to start slowly and gradually increase intensity and duration of practice.

Overall, mind-body techniques can be effective in managing chronic pain. By incorporating mindfulness, meditation, cognitive-behavioural therapy, yoga, or tai chi techniques into their daily routine, individuals with chronic pain can reduce stress, improve their ability to cope with pain, and improve their overall well-being. It is important to work with a healthcare provider or pain management specialist to determine which techniques may be most effective for individual needs.

Explanation of how these techniques can help manage chronic pain and improve mental health

Mind-body techniques, such as mindfulness, meditation, and cognitive-behavioural therapy, can be effective in managing chronic pain and improving mental health in several ways:

1. Reducing stress: Chronic pain can lead to increased levels of stress, which can exacerbate pain and impact mental health. Mind-body techniques can help reduce stress by promoting relaxation, reducing muscle tension, and calming the mind.
2. Changing thought patterns:
   Thought distortions are patterns of thinking that can contribute to negative emotions, anxiety, and stress. These distorted thoughts are often automatic and habitual and can be difficult to recognize and change without intentional effort. Here are a few common types of thought distortions:

- All-or-nothing thinking: This is the tendency to view things in extremes, such as believing that a situation is either completely good or completely bad, with no shades of grey in between.
- Catastrophizing: This is the tendency to imagine the worst-case scenario, even when it's unlikely to happen. Catastrophizing can lead to anxiety and stress.

- Personalization: This is the tendency to take things personally, even when they're not about you. For example, someone not responding to a text message might be interpreted as a personal slight, when in reality, they might just be busy.
- Mind reading: This is the tendency to assume that you know what others are thinking, without actually checking with them. This can lead to misunderstandings and miscommunication.
- Overgeneralization: This is the tendency to apply a negative experience or outcome to all future situations, even if they're not related. For example, if a job interview goes poorly, overgeneralization might lead to the belief that all job interviews will go poorly.
- Filtering: This is the tendency to focus only on the negative aspects of a situation, while ignoring the positive. This can lead to a skewed perception of reality and increased negative emotions.

- Recognizing and challenging thought distortions is an important part of cognitive behavioral therapy (CBT) and other forms of psychotherapy. By identifying and changing these distorted thoughts, individuals can improve their mental health and overall well-being.

Negative thought patterns can increase pain perception and affect mental health. Cognitive-behavioural therapy can help individuals with chronic pain change their negative thought patterns and

beliefs, leading to improved coping skills and reduced pain intensity.
3. Improving coping skills: Chronic pain can be challenging to manage and can impact mental health. Mind-body techniques can help improve coping skills by teaching individuals to accept their pain and manage their symptoms.
4. Promoting relaxation: Mind-body techniques, such as meditation, yoga, and tai chi, can promote relaxation and reduce tension in the body. This can lead to a reduction in pain intensity and an improvement in overall mental health.
5. Enhancing self-awareness: Mind-body techniques, such as mindfulness, can enhance self-awareness and help individuals with chronic pain become more attuned to their physical and emotional experiences. This can help individuals better manage their pain and improve their mental health.

Mind-body techniques can be effective in managing chronic pain and improving mental health by reducing stress, changing negative thought patterns, improving coping skills, promoting relaxation, and enhancing self-awareness. It is important to work with a healthcare provider or pain management specialist to determine which techniques may be most effective for individual needs.

Tips for integrating mind-body techniques into daily life and treatment plans

Integrating mind-body techniques into daily life and treatment plans can be an effective way to manage chronic pain and improve mental health. Here are some tips for integrating these techniques into daily life:

1. Start small: Start with small, achievable goals. For example, you could aim to practice mindfulness for just a few minutes a day or attend one yoga class per week.
2. Make it a habit: Incorporate mind-body techniques into your daily routine as much as possible. For example, you could practice meditation or deep breathing exercises before bed each night.
3. Be patient: Mind-body techniques may take time to show results. Be patient and continue to practice regularly.
4. Seek support: Seek support from a healthcare provider or pain management specialist who can provide guidance and support in integrating mind-body techniques into your treatment plan.
5. Try different techniques: There are many different mind-body techniques to choose from, so try out a few different ones to see which ones work best for you. Some examples include yoga, meditation, tai chi, and cognitive-behavioural therapy.
6. Attend a class or workshop: Consider attending a class or workshop to learn more about mind-body techniques and receive guidance from an instructor.

7. Track progress: Keep track of progress towards your mind-body technique goals. This can help you stay motivated and make adjustments as needed.

Integrating mind-body techniques into daily life and treatment plans can be an effective way to manage chronic pain and improve mental health. By following these tips, individuals with chronic pain can reduce stress, change negative thought patterns, improve coping skills, promote relaxation, and enhance self-awareness.

- Here is an example of a treatment plan that incorporates the advice for improving coping skills:

- Practice mindfulness: The individual will start by practicing mindfulness meditation for 10-15 minutes per day, with the goal of gradually increasing to 20-30 minutes per day over the course of several weeks. They will be encouraged to attend a mindfulness class or use a mindfulness app to help them with their practice.
- Engage in physical activity: The individual will start a walking program for 30 minutes per day, 3-4 times per week, with the goal of gradually increasing to 60 minutes per day, 5-6 times per week over the course of several weeks. They will also be encouraged to try a yoga or Tai Chi class to help improve physical and mental well-being.

- Seek social support: The individual will be encouraged to connect with friends and family members regularly, and to consider joining a chronic pain support group. They will also be encouraged to talk to a mental health professional to help develop additional coping skills and strategies.
- Learn relaxation techniques: The individual will start practicing deep breathing exercises for 5-10 minutes per day, with the goal of gradually increasing to 15-20 minutes per day over the course of several weeks. They will also be encouraged to try progressive muscle relaxation or guided imagery to help manage stress and anxiety.
- Focus on positive thinking: The individual will start practicing positive affirmations each day and will work with a mental health professional to identify negative thought patterns and develop strategies for challenging and replacing them with more positive and realistic thoughts.
- Practice self-care: The individual will be encouraged to prioritize self-care activities, such as getting enough sleep, eating a healthy diet, and engaging in hobbies or activities they enjoy.

- The treatment plan will be reviewed regularly with the individual, and adjustments will be made as needed based on their progress and needs. The goal of the treatment plan is to help the individual develop and implement coping skills that will improve their overall well-being and quality of life.

Real-life examples of successful mind-body techniques

There are many examples of successful mind-body techniques that have been shown to be effective in managing chronic pain and improving mental health. Here are a few real-life examples:

1. Mindfulness meditation: A study published in the Journal of Pain found that a mindfulness-based stress reduction program was effective in reducing pain and improving quality of life in individuals with chronic pain.
2. Cognitive-behavioural therapy: A study published in the Journal of Pain found that cognitive-behavioural therapy was effective in reducing pain intensity and improving overall functioning in individuals with chronic pain.
3. Yoga: A study published in the Journal of Pain found that a yoga program was effective in reducing pain and improving mood in individuals with chronic low back pain.
4. Tai chi: A study published in the Journal of Rheumatology found that a tai chi program was effective in reducing pain and improving physical function in individuals with knee osteoarthritis.
5. Relaxation techniques: A study published in the Journal of Psychosomatic Research found that relaxation techniques, such as deep breathing and progressive muscle relaxation, were effective in

reducing pain and improving quality of life in individuals with chronic pain.

There are many real-life examples of successful mind-body techniques that can be effective in managing chronic pain and improving mental health. It is important to work with a healthcare provider or pain management specialist to determine which techniques may be most effective for individual needs.

# Chapter 5 Coping Strategies

Strategies for coping with the emotional and psychological impact of chronic pain

Chronic pain can have a significant emotional and psychological impact on individuals, leading to anxiety, depression, and other mental health issues. Here are some strategies for coping with the emotional and psychological impact of chronic pain:

1. Seek support: Reach out to friends, family, or a mental health professional for support. Talking about your feelings can help you feel less isolated and more supported.

2. Practice self-care: Make time for activities that bring you joy and relaxation, such as reading, listening to music, or taking a bath. This can help reduce stress and improve your mood.
3. Engage in positive thinking: Try to focus on positive aspects of your life, such as hobbies, relationships, and personal accomplishments. This can help you maintain a positive outlook and improve your mood.
4. Practice mindfulness: Mindfulness practices, such as meditation or deep breathing exercises, can help reduce stress and improve your ability to cope with pain.
5. Stay active: Engage in physical activity, such as walking or swimming, to help improve your mood and reduce stress.
6. Join a support group: Consider joining a support group for individuals with chronic pain. This can provide a supportive community and an opportunity to share experiences and coping strategies.
7. Seek professional help: If you are struggling with depression or anxiety related to chronic pain, seek help from a mental health professional who can provide therapy or medication as needed.

Overall, coping with the emotional and psychological impact of chronic pain can be challenging, but there are strategies that can help. By seeking support, practicing self-care, engaging in positive thinking, practicing mindfulness, staying active, joining a support group, and seeking professional help, individuals with chronic pain can improve their mental health and overall well-being.

There are many strategies for coping with the emotional and psychological impact of chronic pain, and the most effective strategies may vary from person to person. Here are a few additional strategies that may be helpful:

1. Education: Learn as much as you can about your condition and chronic pain in general. Understanding the causes and mechanisms of pain can help reduce fear and anxiety.
2. Relaxation techniques: In addition to mindfulness practices, other relaxation techniques such as progressive muscle relaxation or guided imagery can help reduce stress and improve mood.
3. Expressive writing: Journaling or expressive writing can help individuals with chronic pain express their emotions and reduce stress.
4. Cognitive reframing: Cognitive reframing involves identifying and changing negative thought patterns related to chronic pain. This can help individuals shift their focus from pain to positive aspects of their lives.
5. Gratitude: Practicing gratitude can help individuals with chronic pain focus on positive aspects of their lives and improve their overall well-being.
6. Social support: Building and maintaining a social support network can help individuals with chronic pain feel less isolated and improve their mood.

7. Mind-body practices: In addition to mindfulness, practices such as yoga, tai chi, or qigong can help reduce stress and improve mood.

Ultimately, the most effective strategies for coping with chronic pain will depend on individual needs and preferences. It is important to work with a healthcare provider or pain management specialist to develop a comprehensive treatment plan that addresses both physical and emotional aspects of chronic pain.

Additionally There are many strategies for coping with the emotional and psychological impact of chronic pain, and the most effective strategies may vary from person to person. Here are a few additional strategies that may be helpful:

1. Education: Learn as much as you can about your condition and chronic pain in general. Understanding the causes and mechanisms of pain can help reduce fear and anxiety.
2. Relaxation techniques: In addition to mindfulness practices, other relaxation techniques such as progressive muscle relaxation or guided imagery can help reduce stress and improve mood.
3. Expressive writing: Journaling or expressive writing can help individuals with chronic pain express their emotions and reduce stress.
4. Cognitive reframing: Cognitive reframing involves identifying and changing negative thought patterns related to chronic pain. This

can help individuals shift their focus from pain to positive aspects of their lives.
5. Gratitude: Practicing gratitude can help individuals with chronic pain focus on positive aspects of their lives and improve their overall well-being.
6. Social support: Building and maintaining a social support network can help individuals with chronic pain feel less isolated and improve their mood.
7. Mind-body practices: In addition to mindfulness, practices such as yoga, tai chi, or qigong can help reduce stress and improve mood.

Ultimately, the most effective strategies for coping with chronic pain will depend on individual needs and preferences. It is important to work with a healthcare provider or pain management specialist to develop a comprehensive treatment plan that addresses both physical and emotional aspects of chronic pain.

How to build a support network of family, friends, and healthcare providers

Building a support network of family, friends, and healthcare providers is an important part of managing chronic pain. Here are some tips for building a support network:

1. Communicate openly: Communicate openly with your family and friends about your condition and how it affects your life. Let them know what kind of support you need and how they can help.

2. Join a support group: Join a support group for individuals with chronic pain. This can provide a supportive community and an opportunity to share experiences and coping strategies.
3. Work with a healthcare provider: Work with a healthcare provider or pain management specialist to develop a comprehensive treatment plan that includes both physical and emotional aspects of chronic pain.
4. Educate others: Educate your family and friends about chronic pain and how it affects your life. This can help them better understand your needs and provide more effective support.
5. Consider counselling: Consider seeing a mental health professional who specializes in chronic pain. They can provide additional support and coping strategies.
6. Use technology: Use technology, such as social media or online support groups, to connect with others who are experiencing similar challenges.
7. Take care of yourself: Make time for self-care activities that promote relaxation and reduce stress. This can help you better manage your pain and improve your overall well-being.

Building a support network can take time and effort, but it can be a valuable source of comfort and support for individuals with chronic pain. By communicating openly, joining a support group, working with healthcare providers, educating others, considering counselling, using technology, and taking care of yourself, you can build a strong and effective support network.

Tips for managing stress, anxiety, and depression

Managing stress, anxiety, and depression is important for individuals with chronic pain, as these conditions can exacerbate pain and impact overall well-being. Here are some tips for managing stress, anxiety, and depression:

1. Practice relaxation techniques: Relaxation techniques such as deep breathing, meditation, or progressive muscle relaxation can help reduce stress and improve mood.
2. Engage in physical activity: Physical activity such as walking, yoga, or swimming can help reduce stress and improve mood.
3. Make time for self-care: Make time for activities that bring you joy and relaxation, such as reading, listening to music, or taking a bath. This can help reduce stress and improve your mood.
4. Seek support: Reach out to friends, family, or a mental health professional for support. Talking about your feelings can help you feel less isolated and more supported.
5. Challenge negative thinking: Negative thinking patterns can exacerbate anxiety and depression. Cognitive-behavioural therapy can help individuals with chronic pain change their negative thought patterns and beliefs, leading to improved coping skills and reduced anxiety and depression.

6. Get enough sleep: Getting enough sleep is important for managing stress, anxiety, and depression. Aim for 7-9 hours of sleep per night.
7. Limit alcohol and caffeine: Alcohol and caffeine can exacerbate anxiety and depression. Limit your intake of these substances.
8. Eat a healthy diet: A healthy diet can help reduce inflammation and improve mood. Aim for a diet rich in fruits, vegetables, whole grains, and lean proteins.

Overall, managing stress, anxiety, and depression can be challenging, but there are strategies that can help. By practicing relaxation techniques, engaging in physical activity, making time for self-care, seeking support, challenging negative thinking, getting enough sleep, limiting alcohol and caffeine, and eating a healthy diet, individuals with chronic pain can improve their mental health and overall well-being.

The importance of self-care and self-compassion

Managing stress, anxiety, and depression is important for individuals with chronic pain, as these conditions can exacerbate pain and impact overall well-being. Here are some tips for managing stress, anxiety, and depression:

1. Practice relaxation techniques: Relaxation techniques such as deep breathing, meditation, or progressive muscle relaxation can help reduce stress and improve mood.
2. Engage in physical activity: Physical activity such as walking, yoga, or swimming can help reduce stress and improve mood.
3. Make time for self-care: Make time for activities that bring you joy and relaxation, such as reading, listening to music, or taking a bath. This can help reduce stress and improve your mood.
4. Seek support: Reach out to friends, family, or a mental health professional for support. Talking about your feelings can help you feel less isolated and more supported.
5. Challenge negative thinking: Negative thinking patterns can exacerbate anxiety and depression. Cognitive-behavioural therapy can help individuals with chronic pain change their negative thought patterns and beliefs, leading to improved coping skills and reduced anxiety and depression.
6. Get enough sleep: Getting enough sleep is important for managing stress, anxiety, and depression. Aim for 7-9 hours of sleep per night.
7. Limit alcohol and caffeine: Alcohol and caffeine can exacerbate anxiety and depression. Limit your intake of these substances.
8. Eat a healthy diet: A healthy diet can help reduce inflammation and improve mood. Aim for a diet rich in fruits, vegetables, whole grains, and lean proteins.

Managing stress, anxiety, and depression can be challenging, but there are strategies that can help. By practicing relaxation techniques, engaging in physical activity, making time for self-care, seeking support, challenging negative thinking, getting enough sleep, limiting alcohol and caffeine, and eating a healthy diet, individuals with chronic pain can improve their mental health and overall well-being.

Chronic pain can be a debilitating condition that not only affects an individual's physical health but also their mental and emotional well-being. The constant pain can cause stress, anxiety, and depression, which can further exacerbate the pain and impact an individual's quality of life. Therefore, it is essential to manage stress, anxiety, and depression effectively when dealing with chronic pain. In this article, we will explore some tips for managing stress, anxiety, and depression.

1. Practice relaxation techniques

Relaxation techniques such as deep breathing, meditation, or progressive muscle relaxation can help reduce stress and improve mood. By practicing relaxation techniques, individuals with chronic pain can calm their minds and reduce their physical tension, leading to improved mental and emotional well-being.

Deep breathing involves taking slow, deep breaths through the nose and exhaling slowly through the mouth. This technique can be done anywhere and anytime and can help reduce stress and anxiety.

Meditation involves focusing on a specific object or thought to calm the mind and improve focus. Meditation has been shown to reduce stress, anxiety, and depression in individuals with chronic pain.

Progressive muscle relaxation involves tensing and releasing different muscle groups in the body to reduce tension and stress. This technique can be done sitting or lying down and can help individuals with chronic pain release physical tension and reduce stress.

2. Engage in physical activity

Physical activity such as walking, yoga, or swimming can help reduce stress and improve mood. Exercise releases endorphins, which are natural painkillers that can improve mood and reduce pain.

Individuals with chronic pain should start with low-impact exercises such as walking or swimming and gradually increase the intensity as their condition improves. Exercise can also improve sleep quality, which can further improve mental and emotional well-being.

3. Make time for self-care

Making time for activities that bring joy and relaxation can help reduce stress and improve mood. Individuals with chronic pain should make time for self-care activities such as reading, listening to music, or taking a warm bath.

By making time for self-care, individuals with chronic pain can reduce stress and improve their overall well-being. It is important to find activities that are enjoyable and relaxing to help reduce stress and improve mood.

4. Seek support

Chronic pain can be a lonely and isolating condition. Seeking support from friends, family, or a mental health professional can help individuals with chronic pain feel less isolated and more supported.

Talking about feelings and experiences can help individuals with chronic pain reduce stress and improve their mental and emotional well-being. A mental health professional can provide additional support and coping strategies for managing stress, anxiety, and depression.

5. Challenge negative thinking

Negative thinking patterns can exacerbate anxiety and depression. Cognitive-behavioural therapy (CBT) can help individuals with chronic pain change their negative thought patterns and beliefs, leading to improved coping skills and reduced anxiety and depression.

CBT involves identifying negative thought patterns and beliefs and replacing them with positive, realistic ones. By changing negative thought patterns, individuals with chronic pain can improve their mental and emotional well-being and reduce stress, anxiety, and depression.

6. Get enough sleep

    Adequate sleep is important for individuals suffering from chronic pain because it plays a crucial role in pain management, overall physical and mental health, and quality of life. Here are a few advantages of adequate sleep for individuals with chronic pain:

- Reduces pain intensity: Sleep deprivation can amplify pain intensity and sensitivity, making pain feel more severe. Adequate sleep can help reduce pain intensity and make it easier to manage.
- Improves pain coping mechanisms: Adequate sleep can help individuals develop better coping mechanisms for managing chronic pain. When individuals are well-rested, they may be better equipped to handle stress and pain symptoms.
- Promotes healing: Sleep is a restorative process that helps the body heal and recover from injuries and illnesses. Adequate sleep can help reduce inflammation and promote tissue repair, which can help alleviate pain symptoms.
- Reduces stress and anxiety: Sleep deprivation can contribute to stress and anxiety, which can exacerbate pain symptoms. Adequate sleep can help reduce stress and anxiety, making it easier to manage chronic pain.
- Improves overall physical and mental health: Adequate sleep is important for overall physical and mental health. Chronic pain can lead to sleep disturbances, which can contribute to a range of health problems, including depression, anxiety, and cardiovascular

disease. Adequate sleep can help improve overall health and quality of life.

- It's important for individuals with chronic pain to prioritize sleep hygiene and develop healthy sleep habits. This includes going to bed and waking up at the same time each day, avoiding caffeine and alcohol before bedtime, creating a comfortable sleep environment, and engaging in relaxation techniques before bed. If sleep disturbances persist, it may be helpful to talk to a healthcare professional to identify potential underlying causes and develop a treatment plan.

How does sleep do all this what happens when we are sleeping?

During sleep, the body undergoes a variety of restorative processes that are crucial for overall physical and mental health, including:

- Tissue repair: During deep sleep, the body releases growth hormone, which is important for tissue repair and recovery. This process can help reduce inflammation and promote healing in areas of the body that may be contributing to chronic pain.
- Pain modulation: During sleep, the body produces natural painkillers called endorphins, which can help reduce pain sensations. Inadequate sleep can lead to reduced endorphin production, which can amplify pain intensity and sensitivity.
- Stress reduction: Sleep helps regulate the body's stress response system, which can help reduce stress and anxiety. Chronic pain

can contribute to stress and anxiety, which can exacerbate pain symptoms. Adequate sleep can help individuals manage stress and reduce the impact of chronic pain on their mental health.

- Memory consolidation: Sleep is important for memory consolidation, which can help improve cognitive function and overall mental health. This is particularly important for individuals with chronic pain, who may be at increased risk for cognitive decline and other mental health problems.
- Hormone regulation: Sleep plays a role in regulating hormone production and metabolism, which can impact a range of bodily functions, including appetite, metabolism, and immune function. Adequate sleep can help promote overall physical health and reduce the risk of chronic health problems associated with chronic pain.

Overall, sleep is a critical component of physical and mental health and plays an important role in pain management for individuals with chronic pain. Prioritizing healthy sleep habits and addressing sleep disturbances can help individuals manage chronic pain symptoms and improve overall quality of life.

Getting enough sleep is essential for managing stress, anxiety, and depression. Chronic pain can make it challenging to get enough sleep, but individuals with chronic pain should aim for 7-9 hours of sleep per night.

Creating a sleep-friendly environment, such as a dark, quiet, and cool room, can help individuals with chronic pain improve their sleep quality. It is also important to establish a consistent sleep routine and avoid stimulating activities such as watching television or using electronic devices before bedtime.

7. Limit alcohol and caffeine

Alcohol and caffeine can exacerbate anxiety and depression. Individuals with chronic pain should limit their intake of these substances to improve their mental and emotional well-being.

Chronic pain can be a debilitating condition that not only affects an individual's physical health but also their mental and emotional well-being. The constant pain can cause stress, anxiety, and depression, which can further exacerbate the pain and impact an individual's quality of life. Therefore, it is essential to manage stress, anxiety, and depression effectively when dealing with chronic pain. In this article, we will explore some tips for managing stress, anxiety, and depression.

1. Practice relaxation techniques

Relaxation techniques such as deep breathing, meditation, or progressive muscle relaxation can help reduce stress and improve mood. By practicing relaxation techniques, individuals with chronic pain can calm their minds and reduce their physical tension, leading to improved mental and emotional well-being.

Deep breathing involves taking slow, deep breaths through the nose and exhaling slowly through the mouth. This technique can be done anywhere and anytime and can help reduce stress and anxiety.

Meditation involves focusing on a specific object or thought to calm the mind and improve focus. Meditation has been shown to reduce stress, anxiety, and depression in individuals with chronic pain.

Progressive muscle relaxation involves tensing and releasing different muscle groups in the body to reduce tension and stress. This technique can be done sitting or lying down and can help individuals with chronic pain release physical tension and reduce stress.

2. Engage in physical activity

Physical activity such as walking, yoga, or swimming can help reduce stress and improve mood. Exercise releases endorphins, which are natural painkillers that can improve mood and reduce pain.

Individuals with chronic pain should start with low-impact exercises such as walking or swimming and gradually increase the intensity as their condition improves. Exercise can also improve sleep quality, which can further improve mental and emotional well-being.

3. Make time for self-care

Making time for activities that bring joy and relaxation can help reduce stress and improve mood. Individuals with chronic pain should make time for self-care activities such as reading, listening to music, or taking a warm bath.

By making time for self-care, individuals with chronic pain can reduce stress and improve their overall well-being. It is important to find activities that are enjoyable and relaxing to help reduce stress and improve mood.

4. Seek support

Chronic pain can be a lonely and isolating condition. Seeking support from friends, family, or a mental health professional can help individuals with chronic pain feel less isolated and more supported.

Talking about feelings and experiences can help individuals with chronic pain reduce stress and improve their mental and emotional well-being. A mental health professional can provide additional support and coping strategies for managing stress, anxiety, and depression.

5. Challenge negative thinking

Negative thinking patterns can exacerbate anxiety and depression. Cognitive-behavioural therapy (CBT) can help individuals with chronic pain change their negative thought patterns and beliefs, leading to improved coping skills and reduced anxiety and depression.

CBT involves identifying negative thought patterns and beliefs and replacing them with positive, realistic ones. By changing negative thought patterns, individuals with chronic pain can improve their mental and emotional well-being and reduce stress, anxiety, and depression.

6. Get enough sleep

Getting enough sleep is essential for managing stress, anxiety, and depression. Chronic pain can make it challenging to get enough sleep, but individuals with chronic pain should aim for 7-9 hours of sleep per night.

Creating a sleep-friendly environment, such as a dark, quiet, and cool room, can help individuals with chronic pain improve their sleep quality. It is also important to establish a consistent sleep routine and avoid stimulating activities such as watching television or using electronic devices before bedtime.

7. Limit alcohol and caffeine

Alcohol and caffeine can exacerbate anxiety and depression. Individuals with chronic pain should limit their intake of these substances to improve their mental and emotional well-being.

Alcohol can also interfere with sleep quality, which can further exacerbate stress, anxiety, and depression. Individuals with chronic pain should avoid alcohol or limit their intake to one or two drinks per day.

Caffeine can increase heart rate and blood pressure, leading to increased anxiety and stress. Individuals with chronic pain should limit their intake of caffeine or switch to decaf options to reduce anxiety and stress.

8. Eat a healthy diet

A healthy diet can help reduce inflammation and improve mood. Individuals with chronic pain should aim for a diet rich in fruits, vegetables, whole grains, and lean proteins. A healthy diet can also improve overall health and reduce the risk of chronic diseases such as obesity, diabetes, and heart disease.

In addition to these tips, individuals with chronic pain should work with a healthcare provider or pain management specialist to develop a comprehensive treatment plan that addresses both physical and emotional aspects of chronic pain. This may include medications, physical therapy, alternative therapies, and mental health support.

It is important to remember that managing stress, anxiety, and depression when dealing with chronic pain is a journey and not a quick fix. It takes time, effort, and patience to develop effective coping strategies that work for each individual. However, with the right support, individuals with chronic pain can improve their mental and emotional well-being, reduce stress, anxiety, and depression, and improve their overall quality of life. Inflammation is a natural response of the body's immune system to injury or infection. However, chronic inflammation can contribute to the development of many chronic diseases, including heart disease, cancer, and diabetes. Therefore, it is essential to maintain a healthy anti-inflammatory diet to reduce inflammation and improve overall health.

1. Fruits and vegetables

Fruits and vegetables are rich in antioxidants and anti-inflammatory compounds that can help reduce inflammation and improve overall health. Berries, such as blueberries and raspberries, are particularly high in antioxidants and have been shown to reduce inflammation. Leafy greens, such as kale and spinach, are also rich in antioxidants and anti-inflammatory compounds.

2. Omega-3 fatty acids

Omega-3 fatty acids are essential fatty acids that have anti-inflammatory properties. Fatty fish such as salmon, tuna, and mackerel are high in omega-3 fatty acids. Other sources of omega-3 fatty acids include chia seeds, flaxseeds, and walnuts.

3. Whole grains

Whole grains such as oats, quinoa, and brown rice are high in fibre and have been shown to reduce inflammation. They are also a good source of vitamins and minerals.

4. Lean protein

Lean protein such as chicken, turkey, and fish are low in saturated fats and can help reduce inflammation. Plant-based sources of protein such as beans, lentils, and tofu are also good options.

5. Nuts and seeds

Nuts and seeds such as almonds, cashews, and pumpkin seeds are rich in antioxidants and anti-inflammatory compounds. They are also a good source of healthy fats.

6. Herbs and spices

Herbs and spices such as turmeric, ginger, and cinnamon have anti-inflammatory properties and can help reduce inflammation. Adding these spices to meals can not only improve their flavour but also their health benefits.

7. Healthy fats

Healthy fats such as olive oil, avocado, and nuts are rich in monounsaturated and polyunsaturated fats, which can help reduce inflammation. They are also a good source of vitamins and minerals.

8. Probiotics

Probiotics are beneficial bacteria that live in the gut and have been shown to reduce inflammation. Foods such as yogurt, kefir, and fermented vegetables such as sauerkraut and kimchi are good sources of probiotics.

In addition to incorporating these anti-inflammatory foods into your diet, it is important to avoid foods that can contribute to inflammation. These include:

1. Processed foods

Processed foods such as fast food, chips, and candy are high in sugar, salt, and unhealthy fats, which can contribute to inflammation.

2. Trans fats

Trans fats are found in fried foods, baked goods, and processed snacks. They have been shown to increase inflammation and contribute to chronic diseases.

3. High-glycaemic-index foods

High-glycaemic-index foods such as white bread, pasta, and sugary drinks can cause spikes in blood sugar levels, leading to inflammation.

4. Excessive alcohol

Excessive alcohol consumption can lead to inflammation in the liver and other parts of the body.

5. Red and processed meat

Red and processed meat are high in saturated fats, which can contribute to inflammation.

It is important to maintain a balanced and healthy diet to reduce inflammation and improve overall health. By incorporating anti-inflammatory foods such as fruits and vegetables, omega-3 fatty acids, whole grains, lean protein, nuts and seeds, herbs and spices, and healthy fats into your diet and avoiding inflammatory foods such as processed foods, trans fats, high-glycaemic-index foods, excessive alcohol, and red and processed meat, you can reduce inflammation and improve your overall health.

Here are seven sample daily meal plans, each with approximately 1500 calories, for different diets:

A. Vegan meal plan:

- Breakfast: Vegan protein smoothie with spinach, banana, plant-based protein powder, and almond milk
- Snack: Sliced apple with almond butter
- Lunch: Vegan lentil soup with a side of mixed greens salad topped with roasted vegetables and avocado dressing
- Snack: Vegan yogurt with mixed berries and nuts
- Dinner: Vegan stir-fry with tofu, mixed vegetables, and quinoa
- Dessert: Vegan dark chocolate and sliced banana

B. Vegetarian meal plan:

- Breakfast: Omelette made with two eggs, spinach, tomato, and cheese
- Snack: Sliced cucumber with hummus
- Lunch: Vegetarian chili with a side of mixed greens salad topped with goat cheese and balsamic vinaigrette
- Snack: Greek yogurt with mixed berries and granola
- Dinner: Grilled portobello mushroom burger with avocado and sweet potato fries
- Dessert: Fresh fruit salad with a dollop of whipped cream

C. Carnivore meal plan:

- Breakfast: Three egg omelette with ham, cheese, and mushrooms
- Snack: Beef jerky and mixed nuts

- Lunch: Grilled chicken salad with mixed greens, tomatoes, and balsamic vinaigrette
- Snack: Cheese and crackers
- Dinner: Grilled steak with eggs

D. Keto meal plan:

A.

- Breakfast: Scrambled eggs with bacon and avocado
- Snack: Cheese sticks and olives
- Lunch: Grilled chicken breast with mixed greens and Caesar dressing
- Snack: Keto-friendly smoothie with almond milk, raspberries, and chia seeds
- Dinner: Baked salmon with asparagus and cauliflower rice
- Dessert: Keto-friendly chocolate truffles

B.

- Breakfast: Keto-friendly pancake with almond flour and berries
- Snack: Hardboiled egg and mixed nuts
- Lunch: Grilled shrimp with mixed greens and lemon vinaigrette
- Snack: Keto-friendly smoothie with coconut milk, spinach, and berries

- Dinner: Grilled lamb chops with roasted Brussels sprouts and mashed cauliflower
- Dessert: Keto-friendly cheesecake

G. Mediterranean meal plan:

- Breakfast: Greek yogurt with mixed berries and granola
- Snack: Hummus and sliced bell peppers
- Lunch: Mediterranean quinoa bowl with chickpeas, roasted vegetables, and tzatziki sauce
- Snack: Mixed nuts and olives
- Dinner: Grilled chicken souvlaki with Greek salad and pita bread
- Dessert: Fresh fruit salad with Greek yogurt and honey

H. FODMAPs meal plan:

- Breakfast: Gluten-free oatmeal with lactose-free milk and blueberries
- Snack: Hardboiled egg and sliced cucumber
- Lunch: Grilled chicken with mixed greens and low-FODMAPs dressing
- Snack: Rice cakes with peanut butter and banana
- Dinner: Grilled salmon with roasted carrots and green beans
- Dessert: Low-FODMAPs chocolate brownie.

Note: These sample meal plans are for informational purposes only and should not be taken as medical or dietary advice. Dietary needs and requirements vary from person to person, so it's important to consult with a healthcare professional or registered dietitian before making any significant dietary changes.

# Chapter 6: Advanced Pain Management Techniques

Chronic pain can be a challenging condition to manage, and traditional treatment methods may not always be effective for everyone. Therefore, it is essential to explore advanced pain management techniques that can provide relief for individuals with chronic pain. In this chapter, we will discuss some advanced pain management techniques that can help individuals with chronic pain manage their condition.

1. Interventional pain management

Interventional pain management involves using minimally invasive procedures to treat chronic pain. These procedures include nerve blocks, epidural injections, and radiofrequency ablation. Interventional pain management can be used to treat a variety of chronic pain conditions, including back pain, neck pain, and joint pain.

Nerve blocks involve injecting a local anaesthetic and a steroid into a specific nerve to block pain signals. Epidural injections involve injecting medication into the epidural space around the spinal cord to reduce inflammation and relieve pain. Radiofrequency ablation involves using heat to destroy the nerve fibres that are causing pain.

Interventional pain management can provide targeted pain relief and may be more effective than traditional treatment methods for some individuals with chronic pain.

2. Neuromodulation

Neuromodulation involves using electrical or magnetic impulses to modulate the nervous system and reduce pain. This technique includes spinal cord stimulation, peripheral nerve stimulation, and deep brain stimulation.

Spinal cord stimulation involves implanting electrodes in the spinal cord that deliver electrical impulses to the nerves, blocking pain signals. Peripheral nerve stimulation involves implanting electrodes near the affected nerves to provide pain relief. Deep brain stimulation involves implanting electrodes in the brain to block pain signals.

Neuromodulation can provide long-term pain relief for individuals with chronic pain who have not responded to traditional treatment methods.

3. Biofeedback

Biofeedback involves using sensors to monitor physiological processes such as muscle tension, heart rate, and skin temperature. This technique can help individuals with chronic pain learn to control their physiological responses to pain and reduce their pain levels.

Biofeedback training typically involves using relaxation techniques such as deep breathing and progressive muscle relaxation while monitoring physiological responses. Over time, individuals with chronic pain can learn to control their physiological responses and reduce their pain levels.

4. Mindfulness-based stress reduction (MBSR)

MBSR involves using mindfulness meditation and yoga to reduce stress and anxiety and improve well-being. This technique can be beneficial for individuals with chronic pain, as stress and anxiety can exacerbate pain levels.

MBSR training typically involves attending weekly sessions where individuals with chronic pain learn mindfulness meditation and yoga techniques. Over time, individuals with chronic pain can learn to use these techniques to reduce stress and anxiety and improve their well-being.

5. Cognitive-behavioural therapy (CBT)

CBT involves identifying negative thought patterns and beliefs and replacing them with positive, realistic ones. This technique can help individuals with chronic pain develop coping strategies for managing pain and improve their overall well-being.

CBT training typically involves attending weekly sessions with a mental health professional who specializes in pain management. Over time, individuals with chronic pain can learn to use CBT techniques to develop effective coping strategies for managing pain and improving their overall well-being.

Advanced pain management techniques such as interventional pain management, neuromodulation, biofeedback, MBSR, and CBT can provide relief for individuals with chronic pain who have not responded to traditional treatment methods. These techniques can provide targeted pain relief and improve overall well-being, reducing stress, anxiety, and depression. It is essential to work with a healthcare provider or pain management specialist to determine which advanced pain management techniques may be most effective for each individual's unique needs.

Explanation of advanced pain management techniques such as nerve blocks, spinal cord stimulation, and infusion therapy

Chronic pain can be a debilitating condition that affects every aspect of an individual's life. When traditional pain management approaches, such as medication and physical therapy, are not effective, advanced pain management techniques may be necessary. These techniques can include nerve blocks, spinal cord stimulation, and infusion therapy.

1. Nerve Blocks

Nerve blocks involve injecting a local anaesthetic and a steroid into a specific nerve or group of nerves to block pain signals. By numbing the area, nerve blocks can provide targeted pain relief for individuals with chronic pain who have not responded to traditional treatment methods. There are several different types of nerve blocks, including:

- Epidural nerve blocks: This type of nerve block involves injecting medication into the epidural space around the spinal cord to reduce inflammation and relieve pain. Epidural nerve blocks can be used to treat chronic pain conditions such as back pain, neck pain, and sciatica.
- Facet joint nerve blocks: This type of nerve block involves injecting medication into the facet joints of the spine to relieve pain. Facet joint nerve blocks can be used to treat chronic pain conditions such as arthritis and spinal stenosis.
- Sympathetic nerve blocks: This type of nerve block involves injecting medication into the sympathetic nerves, which are responsible for regulating blood flow and sweating. Sympathetic nerve blocks can be used to treat chronic pain conditions such as complex regional pain syndrome (CRPS) and reflex sympathetic dystrophy (RSD).

Nerve blocks can provide targeted pain relief for individuals with chronic pain who have not responded to traditional treatment methods.

2. Spinal Cord Stimulation

Spinal cord stimulation involves implanting electrodes in the spinal cord that deliver electrical impulses to the nerves, blocking pain signals. The electrodes are connected to a small device that is implanted under the skin in the abdominal or buttock area. The device sends electrical impulses to the nerves, blocking pain signals and reducing pain levels. Spinal cord stimulation can be used to treat chronic pain conditions such as back pain, neck pain, and nerve pain.

Spinal cord stimulation is typically used when other pain management approaches have failed. It is a minimally invasive procedure that is performed under local anaesthesia. The patient is awake during the procedure and can provide feedback to the surgeon to ensure that the electrodes are placed in the correct location.

3. Infusion Therapy

Infusion therapy involves delivering medication directly into the bloodstream through an IV. Infusion therapy can provide targeted pain relief for individuals with chronic pain who have not responded to traditional treatment methods. There are several different types of infusion therapy, including:

- Intravenous (IV) opioids: This type of medication can be used to relieve severe pain. IV opioids are typically reserved for individuals who have not responded to other pain management approaches.
- Lidocaine infusion: This type of medication can be used to treat nerve pain. Lidocaine infusion is typically used when other pain management approaches have failed.
- Ketamine infusion: This type of medication can be used to treat chronic pain conditions such as CRPS and fibromyalgia. Ketamine infusion is typically used when other pain management approaches have failed.

Infusion therapy is typically administered in an outpatient setting under the supervision of a healthcare provider or pain management specialist.

In conclusion, advanced pain management techniques such as nerve blocks, spinal cord stimulation, and infusion therapy can provide targeted pain relief for individuals with chronic pain who have not responded to traditional treatment methods. These techniques can provide long-term pain relief and improve overall well-being, reducing stress, anxiety, and depression. It is essential to work with a healthcare provider or pain management specialist to determine which advanced pain management techniques may be most effective for each individual's unique needs

How these techniques can be used to manage chronic pain

Chronic pain is a complex condition that affects millions of people worldwide. It can be caused by a variety of factors, such as injury, illness, or surgery, and can significantly impact an individual's quality of life. Traditional pain management approaches, such as medication and physical therapy, are often ineffective in managing chronic pain. In these cases, advanced pain management techniques such as nerve blocks, spinal cord stimulation, and infusion therapy may be necessary to provide targeted pain relief.

1. Nerve Blocks

Nerve blocks involve injecting a local anaesthetic and a steroid into a specific nerve or group of nerves to block pain signals. Nerve blocks can be used to treat a variety of chronic pain conditions, including back pain, neck pain, and joint pain. Epidural nerve blocks, facet joint nerve blocks, and sympathetic nerve blocks are all examples of nerve blocks that can be used to manage chronic pain.

Epidural nerve blocks are commonly used to manage chronic back pain. The medication is injected into the epidural space around the spinal cord, reducing inflammation and relieving pain. Facet joint nerve blocks are commonly used to manage chronic neck and back pain caused by arthritis or spinal stenosis. The medication is injected into the facet joints of the spine, reducing inflammation and relieving pain. Sympathetic nerve blocks are commonly used to manage chronic pain conditions such as CRPS and

RSD. The medication is injected into the sympathetic nerves, blocking pain signals, and reducing pain levels.

Nerve blocks can provide targeted pain relief for individuals with chronic pain who have not responded to traditional treatment methods. They can also be used to diagnose the source of the pain.

2. Spinal Cord Stimulation

Spinal cord stimulation involves implanting electrodes in the spinal cord that deliver electrical impulses to the nerves, blocking pain signals. Spinal cord stimulation can be used to manage chronic pain conditions such as back pain, neck pain, and nerve pain. It is typically used when other pain management approaches have failed.

Spinal cord stimulation is a minimally invasive procedure that is performed under local anaesthesia. The patient is awake during the procedure and can provide feedback to the surgeon to ensure that the electrodes are placed in the correct location. The device is implanted under the skin in the abdominal or buttock area, and the electrodes are implanted near the spinal cord. The device sends electrical impulses to the nerves, blocking pain signals and reducing pain levels.

Spinal cord stimulation can provide long-term pain relief for individuals with chronic pain who have not responded to traditional treatment methods. It can also improve overall well-being, reducing stress, anxiety, and depression.

3. Infusion Therapy

Infusion therapy involves delivering medication directly into the bloodstream through an IV. Infusion therapy can be used to manage chronic pain conditions such as CRPS, fibromyalgia, and nerve pain. There are several different types of infusion therapy, including IV opioids, lidocaine infusion, and ketamine infusion.

IV opioids are typically reserved for individuals who have not responded to other pain management approaches. Lidocaine infusion can be used to treat nerve pain and is typically used when other pain management approaches have failed. Ketamine infusion can be used to manage chronic pain conditions such as CRPS and fibromyalgia and is typically used when other pain management approaches have failed.

Infusion therapy is typically administered in an outpatient setting under the supervision of a healthcare provider or pain management specialist. It can provide targeted pain relief for individuals with chronic pain who have not responded to traditional treatment methods.

In conclusion, advanced pain management techniques such as nerve blocks, spinal cord stimulation, and infusion therapy can be used to manage chronic pain conditions that have not responded to traditional

treatment methods. These techniques can provide targeted pain relief and improve overall well-being, reducing stress, anxiety, and depression. It is essential to
work with a healthcare provider or pain management specialist to determine which advanced pain management techniques may be most effective for each individual's unique needs.

These techniques can be used alone or in combination with other pain management approaches to provide long-term pain relief. They can also help individuals with chronic pain reduce their dependence on medication, which can have adverse side effects and increase the risk of addiction.

It is important to note that advanced pain management techniques are not suitable for everyone. Individuals with certain medical conditions, such as heart disease or bleeding disorders, may not be candidates for these procedures. Additionally, these procedures may not be effective for everyone.

Before considering advanced pain management techniques, individuals should exhaust all other pain management approaches, including medication, physical therapy, and lifestyle changes. They should also have a thorough understanding of the risks and benefits of each technique and work closely with a healthcare provider or pain management specialist to determine the best approach for their individual needs.

In summary, advanced pain management techniques such as nerve blocks, spinal cord stimulation, and infusion therapy can provide targeted pain relief for individuals with chronic pain who have not responded to traditional treatment methods. These techniques can improve overall well-being, reduce stress, anxiety, and depression, and help individuals reduce their dependence on medication. It is important to work with a healthcare provider or pain management specialist to determine which advanced pain management techniques may be most effective for each individual's unique needs.

What to expect during advanced pain management procedures
Advanced pain management procedures, such as nerve blocks, spinal cord stimulation, and infusion therapy, can provide targeted pain relief for individuals with chronic pain who have not responded to traditional treatment methods. Before undergoing these procedures, it is important to understand what to expect during the process.

1. Nerve Blocks

During a nerve block, the patient lies on their stomach or back, and the healthcare provider cleans the skin and applies a local anaesthetic to numb the area. Using imaging guidance, the healthcare provider then inserts a needle into the targeted nerve or group of nerves and injects a local anaesthetic and a steroid. The procedure typically takes between 15 and 30 minutes and can provide immediate pain relief. After the procedure, the patient may experience temporary numbness or weakness in the affected area.

2. Spinal Cord Stimulation

Spinal cord stimulation is typically performed in two stages. During the trial stage, the healthcare provider implants a temporary electrode in the spinal cord through a needle inserted into the epidural space. The patient then uses a handheld remote control to adjust the level of electrical stimulation to find the most effective setting. The trial period typically lasts between 5 and 7 days.

If the trial is successful, the patient returns for the permanent implantation. During this stage, the healthcare provider implants the permanent electrodes in the spinal cord through a small incision made in the back. The patient is under sedation or general anaesthesia during the procedure. Once the electrodes are in place, the healthcare provider connects them to a small device implanted under the skin in the abdominal or buttock area. The device sends electrical impulses to the nerves, blocking pain signals and reducing pain levels.

3. Infusion Therapy

During infusion therapy, the patient receives medication through an IV in an outpatient setting. The healthcare provider may monitor the patient's blood pressure, heart rate, and breathing during the procedure. The patient may experience temporary side effects, such as nausea, dizziness, or light-headedness, but these typically subside after the procedure is complete.

Before undergoing any advanced pain management procedure, it is important to discuss the risks and benefits with a healthcare provider or pain management specialist. The patient may need to undergo a series of diagnostic tests, such as MRI or CT scans, to determine the source of the pain and the most appropriate treatment approach.

In conclusion, advanced pain management procedures can provide targeted pain relief for individuals with chronic pain who have not responded to traditional treatment methods. It is important to understand what to expect during these procedures, and to work closely with a healthcare provider or pain management specialist to determine the most appropriate treatment approach.

Potential risks and benefits of advanced pain management techniques

Advanced pain management techniques, such as nerve blocks, spinal cord stimulation, and infusion therapy, can provide targeted pain relief for individuals with chronic pain who have not responded to traditional treatment methods. However, as with any medical procedure, there are potential risks and benefits to consider before undergoing these techniques.

1. Nerve Blocks

Potential Benefits:

- Immediate pain relief: Nerve blocks can provide immediate pain relief, allowing individuals with chronic pain to resume daily activities with less discomfort.
- Targeted pain relief: Nerve blocks target specific nerves or groups of nerves, allowing for more precise pain management than traditional pain medications.
- Reduced dependence on medication: Nerve blocks can provide long-lasting pain relief, reducing the need for daily pain medication.
- Improved quality of life: Reduced pain levels can improve overall well-being, reducing stress, anxiety, and depression.

Potential Risks:

- Nerve damage: While rare, there is a risk of nerve damage during a nerve block procedure. This can result in temporary or permanent numbness or weakness in the affected area.
- Infection: There is a risk of infection at the injection site.
- Bleeding: There is a risk of bleeding at the injection site, particularly for individuals taking blood-thinning medications.

- Allergic reaction: There is a risk of an allergic reaction to the local anaesthetic or steroid used during the procedure.
2. Spinal Cord Stimulation

Potential Benefits:

- Long-term pain relief: Spinal cord stimulation can provide long-lasting pain relief for individuals with chronic pain who have not responded to traditional treatment methods.
- Reduced dependence on medication: Spinal cord stimulation can reduce the need for daily pain medication, reducing the risk of adverse side effects and addiction.
- Improved quality of life: Reduced pain levels can improve overall well-being, reducing stress, anxiety, and depression.

Potential Risks:

- Infection: There is a risk of infection at the site of the implantation or along the leads.
- Bleeding: There is a risk of bleeding during the implantation procedure or along the leads.
- Hardware malfunction: There is a risk of hardware malfunction, such as lead migration or device failure.
- Allergic reaction: There is a risk of an allergic reaction to the materials used in the device.
3. Infusion Therapy

Potential Benefits:

- Targeted pain relief: Infusion therapy delivers medication directly into the bloodstream, providing targeted pain relief.
- Reduced dependence on medication: Infusion therapy can reduce the need for daily pain medication, reducing the risk of adverse side effects and addiction.
- Improved quality of life: Reduced pain levels can improve overall well-being, reducing stress, anxiety, and depression.

Potential Risks:

- Infection: There is a risk of infection at the site of the IV insertion.
- Bleeding: There is a risk of bleeding at the site of the IV insertion, particularly for individuals taking blood-thinning medications.
- Allergic reaction: There is a risk of an allergic reaction to the medication used during the procedure.
- Organ damage: Infusion therapy can cause damage to the liver, kidneys, or other organs over time.

It is important to discuss the risks and benefits of advanced pain management techniques with a healthcare provider or pain management specialist before undergoing any procedure. It is also important to understand that not all individuals with chronic pain will be suitable candidates for these techniques, and that alternative approaches may be more appropriate.

Advanced pain management techniques such as nerve blocks, spinal cord stimulation, and infusion therapy can provide targeted pain relief for individuals with chronic pain who have not responded to traditional treatment methods. While there are potential risks to consider, the potential benefits can include long-lasting pain relief, reduced dependence on medication, and improved quality of life. It is important to work closely with a healthcare provider or pain management specialist to determine

When considering the potential risks and benefits of advanced pain management techniques, it is important to take into account the individual's medical history, current health status, and overall treatment goals.

For example, individuals with a history of allergies or previous complications during medical procedures may be at higher risk for adverse reactions during nerve blocks, spinal cord stimulation, or infusion therapy. Additionally, individuals with certain medical conditions, such as heart disease or bleeding disorders, may not be candidates for these procedures due to the increased risk of complications.

It is also important to consider the potential benefits of advanced pain management techniques beyond pain relief. For example, reduced pain levels can improve overall well-being, reducing stress, anxiety, and depression. This can have a positive impact on other aspects of an individual's life, such as work productivity, social relationships, and quality of sleep.

However, it is also important to understand that advanced pain management techniques are not suitable for everyone and may not provide the same level of pain relief for all individuals. It is important to work with a healthcare provider or pain management specialist to determine the most appropriate treatment approach for each individual's unique needs.

Additionally, individuals undergoing advanced pain management techniques should be closely monitored for any potential complications, such as infection, bleeding, or hardware malfunction. This may involve regular check-ups with a healthcare provider or pain management specialist, as well as ongoing monitoring of the device or medication used.

In summary, when considering the potential risks and benefits of advanced pain management techniques, it is important to take into account the individual's medical history, current health status, and overall treatment goals. While these techniques can provide targeted pain relief and improve overall well-being, it is important to work closely with a healthcare provider or pain management specialist to determine the most appropriate treatment approach and closely monitor for any potential complications.

# Chapter 7 Strategies for Long-Term Success

Managing chronic pain is an ongoing process that requires long-term commitment and dedication. Once an individual has established a treatment plan that provides effective pain management, it is important to focus on maintaining progress and continuing to manage chronic pain in the long term.

1. Follow-Up Care

Regular follow-up care with a healthcare provider or pain management specialist is essential for monitoring progress and making any necessary adjustments to the treatment plan. This may involve regular check-ups, diagnostic tests, and ongoing assessments of pain levels and medication effectiveness.

2. Healthy Lifestyle Habits

Adopting healthy lifestyle habits, such as regular exercise, a balanced diet, and adequate sleep, can help improve overall well-being and reduce stress, anxiety, and depression. These habits can also help manage chronic pain by reducing inflammation, improving joint mobility, and reducing pressure on the nerves.

3. Stress Management Techniques

Stress and anxiety can exacerbate chronic pain, so it is important to adopt stress management techniques such as meditation, deep breathing exercises, and relaxation techniques to reduce stress levels. Cognitive-behavioural therapy (CBT) can also be helpful in developing coping strategies for dealing with stress and anxiety.

4. Mind-Body Techniques

Mind-body techniques, such as mindfulness, meditation, and yoga, can help manage chronic pain by reducing stress levels and improving overall well-being. These techniques can also help individuals develop a greater awareness of their body and pain sensations, allowing them to manage pain more effectively.

5. Social Support

Having a strong support network of family, friends, and healthcare providers can be crucial in managing chronic pain in the long term. Support from others can provide emotional support, practical assistance, and motivation to stick with a treatment plan and maintain progress.

6. Pain Management Tools

Using pain management tools such as heat or ice packs, massage, or transcutaneous electrical nerve stimulation (TENS) can also be helpful in managing chronic pain in the long term. These tools can provide temporary relief and complement other pain management strategies.

7. Avoiding Triggers

Identifying and avoiding triggers that exacerbate chronic pain can help individuals maintain progress and manage pain in the long term. Triggers may include certain foods, activities, or environmental factors that increase pain levels.

In summary, maintaining progress and managing chronic pain in the long term requires a multi-faceted approach that includes regular follow-up care, healthy lifestyle habits, stress management techniques, mind-body techniques, social support, pain management tools, and avoiding triggers. It is important to work closely with a healthcare provider or pain management specialist to develop a long-term treatment plan that meets the individual's unique needs and supports ongoing pain management. How do you avoid triggers?

Avoiding triggers can be an effective strategy for managing chronic pain in the long term. Here are some tips for identifying and avoiding triggers:

1. Keep a Pain Journal

Keeping a pain journal can help individuals identify patterns or triggers that exacerbate their chronic pain. In the journal, individuals should note their pain levels, activities, foods, and environmental factors that may have contributed to the pain.

2. Identify Triggers

Once patterns have been identified, individuals should work with a healthcare provider or pain management specialist to identify specific triggers that may be exacerbating their chronic pain. Triggers may include certain foods, activities, or environmental factors.

3. Modify Your Environment

Modifying the environment to reduce exposure to triggers can be an effective strategy for managing chronic pain. For example, if noise exacerbates pain, wearing earplugs or using noise-cancelling headphones can help reduce pain levels. If bright lights are a trigger, wearing sunglasses or using curtains to block out light can help.

4. Make Lifestyle Changes

Making lifestyle changes, such as adopting a healthy diet, regular exercise, and good sleep hygiene, can also help reduce the impact of triggers on chronic pain. For example, if certain foods exacerbate pain, individuals may consider modifying their diet to avoid those foods.

5. Develop Coping Strategies

Developing coping strategies for managing triggers can also be helpful in managing chronic pain in the long term. This may include deep breathing exercises, meditation, or other relaxation techniques.

6. Seek Support

Having a strong support network can also be helpful in managing triggers and chronic pain. Friends, family, or support groups can provide emotional support, practical assistance, and motivation to stick with a treatment plan and manage pain effectively.

In summary, avoiding triggers is an important strategy for managing chronic pain in the long term. This involves identifying triggers, modifying the environment, making lifestyle changes, developing coping strategies, and seeking support. Working closely with a healthcare provider or pain management specialist can help individuals identify and manage triggers effectively.

So what are coping strategies?

Coping strategies refer to the different techniques and tools individuals can use to manage chronic pain and its associated challenges. Here are some examples of coping strategies:

1. Relaxation Techniques

Relaxation techniques, such as deep breathing exercises, progressive muscle relaxation, and guided imagery, can help reduce stress levels and alleviate pain.

2. Mind-Body Techniques

Mind-body techniques, such as mindfulness meditation, yoga, and tai chi, can help manage chronic pain by improving mood, reducing stress levels, and enhancing overall well-being.

3. Cognitive-Behavioural Therapy

Cognitive-behavioural therapy (CBT) is a form of psychotherapy that can help individuals identify and change negative thought patterns and behaviours that may contribute to their chronic pain.

4. Pain Management Tools

Pain management tools, such as heat or ice packs, massage, or transcutaneous electrical nerve stimulation (TENS), can provide temporary relief from pain and complement other pain management strategies.

5. Social Support

Having a strong support network of family, friends, and healthcare providers can provide emotional support, practical assistance, and motivation to stick with a treatment plan and manage pain effectively.

6. Time Management

Managing time effectively can help reduce stress levels and alleviate pain. This may involve prioritizing activities and delegating tasks, taking breaks throughout the day, and pacing activities to avoid overexertion.

7. Positive Thinking

Maintaining a positive outlook and focusing on things that bring joy and happiness can help improve mood and reduce stress levels, which can in turn help manage chronic pain.

8. Self-Care

Taking care of oneself, both physically and emotionally, can help manage chronic pain. This may involve getting adequate sleep, eating a healthy diet, engaging in physical activity, and participating in activities that bring joy and fulfillment.

In summary, coping strategies are different techniques and tools individuals can use to manage chronic pain and its associated challenges. These strategies can help reduce stress levels, improve mood, and enhance overall well-being, allowing individuals to manage their chronic pain more effectively.

How can you identify triggers?

Identifying triggers is an important step in managing chronic pain. Here are some tips for identifying triggers:

1. Keep a Pain Journal

Keeping a pain journal can help individuals identify patterns or triggers that exacerbate their chronic pain. In the journal, individuals should note their pain levels, activities, foods, and environmental factors that may have contributed to the pain.

2. Monitor Daily Activities

Monitoring daily activities can also help individuals identify triggers that exacerbate chronic pain. This may involve paying attention to activities such as standing for long periods, sitting in one position, or lifting heavy objects.

3. Consider Emotional Triggers

Emotional triggers, such as stress, anxiety, and depression, can also exacerbate chronic pain. Individuals should consider how their emotional state may be contributing to their pain.

4. Think About Environmental Factors

Environmental factors, such as noise, bright lights, and temperature changes, can also trigger chronic pain. Individuals should consider how their environment may be contributing to their pain.

5. Identify Food Triggers

Certain foods may trigger chronic pain, particularly if an individual has a food sensitivity or allergy. Identifying these food triggers and avoiding them can help manage chronic pain.

6. Seek Professional Help

Working with a healthcare provider or pain management specialist can also help individuals identify triggers and develop a plan for managing chronic pain. A healthcare provider may be able to conduct diagnostic tests or provide guidance on managing pain triggers.

In summary, identifying triggers is an important step in managing chronic pain. Keeping a pain journal, monitoring daily activities, considering emotional and environmental factors, identifying food triggers, and seeking professional help can all help individuals identify triggers and develop a plan for managing chronic pain.

What is the most effective plan for modifying your environment?

Modifying the environment can be an effective strategy for managing chronic pain. Here are some tips for creating a pain-friendly environment:

1. Reduce Noise

Excess noise can be a trigger for chronic pain. To reduce noise levels, individuals may use noise-cancelling headphones, earplugs, or sound machines.

2. Control Lighting

Bright or flickering lights can also trigger chronic pain. Using curtains or shades to block out bright light, avoiding fluorescent lights, and using low-wattage bulbs can help reduce pain.

3. Adjust Temperature

Extreme temperatures can also exacerbate chronic pain. Keeping the environment at a comfortable temperature, using a space heater or fan, and dressing appropriately can help manage pain.

4. Use Supportive Furniture

Supportive furniture, such as chairs with lumbar support or adjustable desks, can help reduce pressure on the spine and joints, reducing pain levels.

5. Reduce Clutter

A cluttered environment can be overwhelming and contribute to stress levels. Reducing clutter and organizing the space can help promote relaxation and reduce pain levels.

6. Create a Comfortable Sleep Environment

A comfortable sleep environment can help improve sleep quality and reduce pain levels. This may involve investing in a comfortable mattress and pillows, using supportive bedding, and using a white noise machine.

7. Use Assistive Devices

Assistive devices, such as grab bars, shower chairs, and mobility aids, can help reduce the risk of falls and promote safety and independence, reducing pain levels.

In summary, modifying the environment can be an effective strategy for managing chronic pain. Reducing noise, controlling lighting, adjusting temperature, using supportive furniture, reducing clutter, creating a comfortable sleep environment, and using assistive devices can all help create a pain-friendly environment. Working with a healthcare provider or pain management specialist can also help individuals identify environmental factors that may contribute to their chronic pain and develop a plan for managing pain triggers.

Understanding how to maintain progress and continue managing chronic pain in the long term

Managing chronic pain in the long term can be challenging, but there are several strategies that can help individuals maintain progress and continue to manage their pain effectively. Here are some tips for managing chronic pain in the long term:

1. Stick to Your Treatment Plan

Consistently following a treatment plan can help individuals manage chronic pain in the long term. This may involve taking medication as prescribed, attending physical therapy or other appointments, and practicing coping strategies regularly.

2. Monitor Your Progress

Monitoring progress can help individuals identify what is working and what needs to be modified in their treatment plan. Keeping a pain journal, tracking changes in pain levels, and evaluating the effectiveness of different strategies can help individuals make informed decisions about managing their pain.

3. Continue to Learn About Pain Management

Staying informed about pain management can help individuals stay up to date with new treatment options and strategies. This may involve attending workshops, reading books or articles, or seeking guidance from healthcare providers or pain management specialists.

4. Engage in Regular Physical Activity

Regular physical activity can help manage chronic pain in the long term. Engaging in activities such as walking, swimming, or yoga can help improve flexibility, reduce stress, and alleviate pain.

5. Practice Self-Care

Taking care of oneself, both physically and emotionally, is important for managing chronic pain in the long term. This may involve getting adequate sleep, eating a healthy diet, engaging in activities that bring joy and fulfillment, and practicing relaxation techniques.

6. Seek Support

Having a strong support network can also be helpful in managing chronic pain in the long term. Friends, family, or support groups can provide emotional support, practical assistance, and motivation to stick with a treatment plan and manage pain effectively.

7. Set Realistic Goals

Setting realistic goals can help individuals stay motivated and maintain progress in managing chronic pain. Goals should be specific, measurable, and achievable.

In summary, managing chronic pain in the long term requires consistent effort and a variety of strategies. Sticking to a treatment plan, monitoring progress, continuing to learn about pain management, engaging in regular physical activity, practicing self-care, seeking support, and setting realistic goals can all help individuals maintain progress and continue managing their chronic pain effectively.

Strategies for preventing relapse and managing setbacks

Managing chronic pain can be a long-term process that involves many ups and downs. Setbacks and relapses are common and can be discouraging, but there are several strategies that can help individuals prevent relapse and manage setbacks. Here are some tips for preventing relapse and managing setbacks:

1. Identify Triggers

Identifying triggers is an important step in preventing relapse and managing setbacks. Keeping a pain journal, monitoring daily activities, considering emotional and environmental factors, identifying food triggers, and seeking professional help can all help individuals identify triggers that may contribute to relapse.

2. Develop Coping Strategies

Coping strategies can help individuals manage pain during setbacks and prevent relapse. Relaxation techniques, mind-body techniques, cognitive behavioral therapy, pain management tools, social support, time management, positive thinking, and self-care are all coping strategies that can be helpful during setbacks.

3. Stick to a Treatment Plan

Sticking to a treatment plan is important for preventing relapse and managing setbacks. Consistently following a treatment plan can help individuals manage pain effectively and avoid relapse.

4. Stay Active

Staying active is important for managing chronic pain and preventing relapse. Engaging in physical activity, such as walking, swimming, or yoga, can help improve flexibility, reduce stress, and alleviate pain.

5. Monitor Progress

Monitoring progress can help individuals identify what is working and what needs to be modified in their treatment plan. Keeping a pain journal, tracking changes in pain levels, and evaluating the effectiveness of different strategies can help individuals make informed decisions about managing their pain.

6. Seek Support

Having a strong support network can be helpful in managing setbacks and preventing relapse. Friends, family, or support groups can provide emotional support, practical assistance, and motivation to stick with a treatment plan and manage pain effectively.

7. Set Realistic Goals

Setting realistic goals can help individuals stay motivated and maintain progress in managing chronic pain. Goals should be specific, measurable, and achievable.

8. Learn From Setbacks

Setbacks can be frustrating, but they can also provide valuable learning experiences. Analysing setbacks, identifying what went wrong, and making adjustments to the treatment plan can help individuals prevent future relapses and manage setbacks more effectively.

In summary, preventing relapse and managing setbacks requires consistent effort and a variety of strategies. Identifying triggers, developing coping strategies, sticking to a treatment plan, staying active, monitoring progress, seeking support, setting realistic goals, and learning from setbacks can all help individuals prevent relapse and manage setbacks effectively.

Tips for adjusting to life with chronic pain and finding meaning and purpose

Living with chronic pain can be challenging, but there are several strategies that can help individuals adjust to life with chronic pain and find meaning and purpose. Here are some tips:

1. Acceptance

Accepting the reality of chronic pain can be a difficult process, but it is an important step in adjusting to life with chronic pain. This involves acknowledging that the pain is real and that it may be a long-term or permanent part of life. Acceptance does not mean giving up or resigning oneself to a life of suffering, but rather recognizing that the pain is a part of life and finding ways to manage it.

One way to practice acceptance is to focus on the present moment, rather than dwelling on the past or worrying about the future. Mindfulness meditation and other mindfulness practices can help individuals learn to be more present and accepting of their pain. Another way to practice acceptance is to develop a positive attitude and cultivate gratitude for the things in life that are still enjoyable.

2. Focus on Abilities

Focusing on abilities, rather than limitations, can help individuals adjust to life with chronic pain. This may involve identifying activities that can still be enjoyed and pursuing new hobbies or interests. For example, if someone enjoys reading but finds it difficult to hold a book for long periods of time, they may try listening to audiobooks instead. Similarly, if someone enjoys gardening but finds it difficult to kneel or stand for long periods of time, they may try container gardening or using a gardening stool.

Focusing on abilities can also involve finding creative solutions to everyday challenges. For example, someone with chronic pain in their hands may use adaptive devices, such as a jar opener or specialized utensils, to make cooking and eating easier.

3. Create a Support System

Creating a support system can provide emotional support and practical assistance. This may involve seeking support from friends and family, joining support groups, or seeking the help of a mental health professional. It is important to surround oneself with people who are understanding and supportive of the challenges of living with chronic pain.

Support groups can provide a sense of community and a safe space to share experiences and coping strategies. Mental health professionals can help individuals develop coping strategies and manage the emotional impact of chronic pain.

4. Practice Self-Care

Taking care of oneself, both physically and emotionally, is important for adjusting to life with chronic pain. This may involve getting adequate sleep, eating a healthy diet, engaging in activities that bring joy and fulfillment, and practicing relaxation techniques. It is important to prioritize self-care and make it a regular part of daily life.

One important aspect of self-care is getting enough restful sleep. Chronic pain can make it difficult to sleep, but practicing good sleep hygiene, such as creating a relaxing bedtime routine and avoiding screens before bed, can help improve sleep quality. Eating a healthy diet and engaging in regular physical activity can also help improve overall health and reduce pain.

5. Set Realistic Goals

Setting realistic goals can help individuals adjust to life with chronic pain. Goals should be specific, measurable, and achievable. For example, rather than setting a goal to run a marathon, someone with chronic pain may set a goal to walk for 30 minutes each day.

Setting goals can provide a sense of purpose and motivation, but it is important to set goals that are realistic and achievable. Unrealistic goals can lead to frustration and disappointment, which can make it more difficult to manage chronic pain.

6. Develop Resilience

Developing resilience can help individuals adjust to life with chronic pain. Resilience is the ability to adapt to adversity and bounce back from setbacks. Cultivating resilience can help individuals develop a positive attitude and cope with the challenges of living with chronic pain.

One way to develop resilience is to cultivate a growth mindset. This involves viewing challenges as opportunities for growth and learning, rather than as insurmountable obstacles. Practicing mindfulness and other relaxation techniques can also help develop resilience by improving emotional regulation and reducing stress.

It is also important to develop coping strategies for managing pain and other symptoms of chronic pain. This may involve using distraction techniques, such as listening to music or engaging in a hobby, to take the focus off of pain. It may also involve using relaxation techniques, such as deep breathing or progressive muscle relaxation, to reduce tension and pain.

7. Find Meaning and Purpose

Finding meaning and purpose in life can help individuals adjust to life with chronic pain. This may involve pursuing hobbies or interests, volunteering, or setting meaningful goals. When life is focused solely on managing pain, it can feel like there is no purpose or joy. Finding ways to incorporate purpose and joy into life can improve overall well-being and make it easier to manage chronic pain.

Finding meaning and purpose may involve setting goals that align with personal values, such as helping others or pursuing creative endeavours. It may also involve finding ways to give back to the community, such as volunteering or participating in advocacy groups for chronic pain.

Adjusting to life with chronic pain requires a variety of strategies, including acceptance, focusing on abilities, creating a support system, practicing self-care, setting realistic goals, developing resilience, and finding meaning and purpose. By incorporating these strategies into daily life, individuals can learn to live a fulfilling life despite chronic pain.

The importance of resilience and cultivating a positive mindset
Resilience and a positive mindset are important factors in managing chronic pain. Chronic pain can be a challenging condition that affects not only physical health, but also emotional well-being. Coping with chronic pain can be difficult, but developing resilience and a positive mindset can help individuals adapt and manage the condition more effectively.

Resilience is the ability to adapt and recover from adversity and is an important quality for individuals with chronic pain. Coping with chronic pain often involves setbacks and challenges, and developing resilience can help individuals bounce back and stay motivated in the face of these challenges. Resilience can be cultivated through various strategies, such as setting realistic goals, practicing mindfulness and other relaxation techniques, and seeking social support.

A positive mindset involves focusing on the positive aspects of life, even in the face of challenges. It is a way of thinking that can help individuals cope with chronic pain and maintain a sense of hope and optimism. This mindset involves viewing challenges as opportunities for growth and focusing on solutions rather than dwelling on problems.

One way to cultivate a positive mindset is through cognitive-behavioral therapy (CBT), which is a type of talk therapy that helps individuals identify negative thought patterns and develop more positive ways of thinking. CBT can help individuals reframe their thoughts about chronic pain and develop a more positive outlook on life.

Another way to cultivate a positive mindset is through gratitude practice. Practicing gratitude involves focusing on the positive aspects of life and expressing gratitude for them. This can help individuals shift their focus away from pain and towards the positive aspects of life.

A positive mindset and resilience are important for managing chronic pain because they can improve overall well-being and help individuals cope with the challenges of living with chronic pain. They can also help individuals stay motivated and engaged in activities that bring joy and fulfillment.

Resilience and a positive mindset are important factors in managing chronic pain. They can be cultivated through various strategies, such as setting realistic goals, practicing mindfulness and other relaxation techniques, seeking social support, cognitive-behavioral therapy, and gratitude practice. Developing resilience and a positive mindset can help individuals adapt and manage the condition more effectively, leading to improved overall well-being and a better quality of life.

Conclusion:
In conclusion, chronic pain can be a challenging and often debilitating condition, but with the right strategies and mindset, individuals can learn to manage and even thrive despite the pain. This book has provided an overview of chronic pain, including its causes and types, as well as the

various treatment options available. Additionally, the book has highlighted the importance of lifestyle changes, mind-body techniques, and advanced pain management techniques in managing chronic pain.

Furthermore, the book has emphasized the importance of developing resilience, cultivating a positive mindset, and finding meaning and purpose in life when living with chronic pain. These skills and strategies can help individuals adapt and manage the condition more effectively, leading to improved overall well-being and a better quality of life.

Whether you are just beginning your journey with chronic pain or have been managing it for some time, this book is a valuable resource for understanding and managing the condition. By incorporating the strategies and techniques presented in this book, individuals can learn to live a fulfilling life despite the challenges of chronic pain.

Recap of key points and takeaways from the book
Here is a recap of some of the key points and takeaways from this book on managing chronic pain:

1. Chronic pain is a complex condition that affects not only physical health but also emotional well-being.
2. It is important to work with healthcare providers to create a personalized treatment plan that incorporates a variety of

strategies, including medication, physical therapy, and alternative therapies.
3. Lifestyle changes, such as adopting a healthy anti-inflammatory diet, regular exercise, and getting enough sleep, can help manage chronic pain.
4. Mind-body techniques, such as mindfulness, meditation, and cognitive-behavioral therapy, can also be effective in managing chronic pain and improving mental health.
5. Advanced pain management techniques, such as nerve blocks, spinal cord stimulation, and infusion therapy, can be used to manage chronic pain when other treatments are not effective.
6. It is important to develop resilience and a positive mindset when living with chronic pain, as this can help individuals adapt and manage the condition more effectively.
7. Coping strategies, such as identifying triggers, creating a supportive environment, and developing a support network, can help individuals manage chronic pain and prevent relapse.
8. Adjusting to life with chronic pain involves finding meaning and purpose in life, as well as staying engaged in activities that bring joy and fulfillment.

Overall, this book provides a comprehensive overview of chronic pain management, from diagnosis and treatment to advanced pain management techniques and coping strategies. By incorporating these strategies and techniques into their lives, individuals can learn to manage and even thrive despite the challenges of chronic pain.

Final words of encouragement and inspiration for readers to take control of their chronic pain and improve their quality of life.

Ahoy there, my dear readers! As you reach the end of this book, I hope you feel empowered and motivated to take control of your chronic pain and improve your quality of life. Remember, chronic pain can be a formidable opponent, but with the right strategies and mindset, you can conquer it and thrive despite the challenges.

It may seem like an uphill battle but think of it as a grand adventure on the high seas of life. You are the captain of your own ship, and with the right crew and strategies, you can navigate even the roughest waters. Don't be afraid to set your sights on the horizon and pursue your dreams, even with chronic pain as a companion.

Remember, you are not alone in this journey. There are many others who have faced similar challenges and have found ways to manage and overcome chronic pain. So, seek out the support and encouragement of others, whether it's through support groups, online communities, or the friendly creatures of the sea.

Finally, be kind and compassionate to yourself. You are doing your best, and every step forward, no matter how small, is a victory. So, celebrate your successes and learn from your setbacks. And above all, never give up hope. With the right mindset and strategies, you can live a fulfilling and meaningful life, even with chronic pain as a companion.

So, hoist the sails and set sail for the horizon, my dear readers. The adventure awaits! For exercises go to you Tube Channel smashchronicpain.com

Manufactured by Amazon.com.au
Sydney, New South Wales, Australia